NURSING DIAGNOSIS POCKET GUIDE

Neonatal and Pediatric CARE PLANS

SHARON ENNIS AXTON, RN, PNP, MS
Nursing Specialist in Pediatric Pulmonary Nursing
Assistant Professor, Texas Tech University Health Sciences Center, School of Nursing Lubbock, Texas

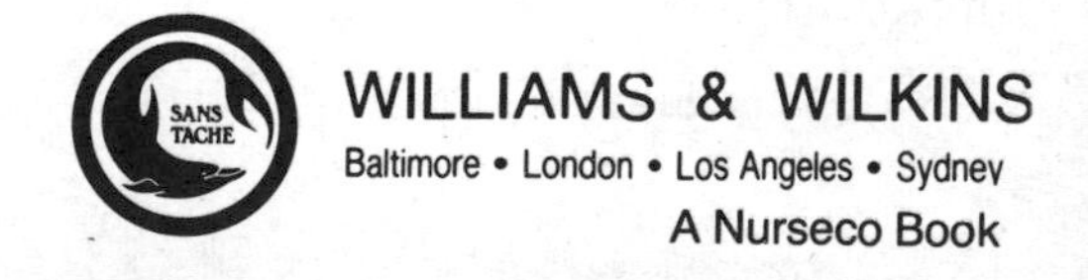

WILLIAMS & WILKINS
Baltimore • London • Los Angeles • Sydney
A Nurseco Book

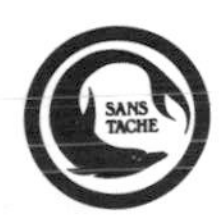

Williams & Wilkins
428 East Preston Street
Baltimore, MD 21202, U.S.A.

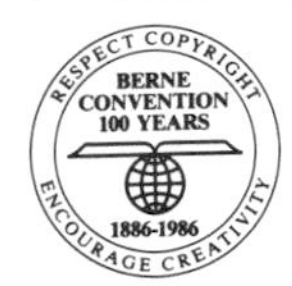

Accurate indications, adverse reactions, and dosage schedules for drugs are provided in this book, but it is possible that they may change. The reader is urged to review the package information data of the manufacturers of the medications mentioned.

Printed in the United States of America
First Edition,

Library of Congress Cataloging in Publication Data

Main entry under title:

Axton, Sharon Ennis.
Neonatal and pediatric nursing care plans.

(Nursing diagnosis pocket guide)
"A Nurseco book."
Bibliography: p.
Includes index.
1. Pediatric nursing. 2. Infants (Newborn)—Diseases—Nursing. 3. Nursing care plans. I. Title. II. Series. [DNLM: 1. Neonatology—handbooks. 2. Neonatology—nurses' instruction. 3. Nursing Process—methods—handbooks. 4. Pediatric Nursing—methods—handbooks. WY 39 A972n]
RJ245.A88 1986 618.92'01 86-4096

Library of Congress Cataloging-in-Publication Data

ISBN 0-683-09508-0

86 87 88 89 90 10 9 8 7 6 5 4 3 2 1

Foreword

The last few years have seen much change in the use of nursing diagnosis by practicing nurses. Nursing diagnosis has moved from being a topic of interest to theorists and teachers to being a part of curriculum and a fact of practice life for many nurses. The work continues. Philosophical concerns are being addressed, diagnoses are undergoing refinement and redefinition, and above all, practicing nurses are becoming more convinced that there is value to the use of diagnoses, both as categories and as reflection of a process of critical thinking about patients' concerns and needs. Nursing has moved from "Do we need nursing diagnosis?" to "How do we use nursing diagnoses?" This book addresses this more recent question while focusing on neonates and children.

The author's perspective that certain nursing diagnoses are predictable when certain pathology is present, is the result of her knowledge of the real world of practice combined with the educator's emphasis on improvement of practice.

This book will help practicing nurses grapple with adding nursing diagnosis to their repertoire. The student who wants a handy reference to augment the basic pediatric test will find this is a useful companion. The faculty member who deals with both students and practicing nurses will find that this book can bridge the distance between ideal and real practice. In sum, it is a fine contribution. That this book delivers what it promises is no surprise when one considers that the author is a nurse specialist whose role encompasses practice, teaching in a health science center school of nursing, scholarly activity, and community service. Fulfilling all those roles requires commitment; **Neonatal and Pediatric Nursing Care Plans** is evidence of that commitment.

Teddy L. Langford, RN, PhD
Dean and Professor
Texas Tech University
Health Sciences Center
School of Nursing

Preface

The impetus to write a book on neonatal and pediatric nursing care plans sprung from my experiences as a practicing nurse and educator. Having students in both neonatal and pediatric clinical settings made it evident that a source was needed to help identify nursing diagnoses for these patients. Many highly skilled and knowledgeable practicing nurses have also expressed a need for such a source.

Although practicing nurses have become familiar with the steps involved in care planning, students are continually learning and refining these steps throughout their education. One of the first steps in developing a nursing care plan is to make a nursing diagnosis. Many good sources are available to aid nurses and students in making *general* nursing diagnoses, however few identify nursing diagnoses for neonatal and pediatric patients. This pocket guide not only identifies the relationship to neonatal and pediatric patients, but also correlates nursing diagnoses with specific medical diagnoses.

The medical diagnoses in **Neonatal and Pediatric Nursing Care Plans** were selected as a result of my experiences as a practicing nurse in both these settings, from reviewing records of hospitalized neonatal and pediatric patients, and from my experiences as a nurse educator.

Most of the nursing diagnoses are those accepted and published by the North American Nursing Diagnosis Association (NANDA). On a few occasions it was necessary to utilize some that have not as yet been approved—these are indicated when they occur.

I would like to express my appreciation to all my colleagues—educators, and practicing nurses—who have influenced me over the years. Special thanks are due to the nursing staff at Lubbock General Hospital, particularly the neonatal and pediatric units, with whom I have most recently had the pleasure of colleagueship.

Contents

Introduction

The goal of **Neonatal and Pediatric Nursing Care Plans** is to assist practicing nurses and students to implement the nursing process for neonatal and pediatric patients. This book provides a quick reference for correlating frequently encountered neonatal and pediatric medical diagnoses with nursing diagnoses.

Each diagnostic entry has a standard set of components:

Medical Diagnosis

Primary Nursing Diagnosis

Definition: This refers only to the nursing diagnosis and not to the medical diagnosis.

Possibly Related to: The rationale for the selection of the primary nursing diagnosis is inherent in this statement.

Characteristics: These are of the selected primary nursing diagnosis *and* of the identified medical diagnosis. The list presents possible signs and symptoms that might be manifested by a child with the identified medical diagnosis.

Expected Outcomes: This is the next step in the nursing process after identification of the nursing diagnosis. They may be listed on a nursing care plan as patient goals, objectives, or planning. Outcomes are written as specifically as possible so they are measurable and can be easily evaluated. Directions are sometimes included to help individualize the expected outcomes for each patient. For example, in the pediatric section, an expected outcome might read as follows:

> Child will have adequate cardiac output as evidenced by:
>
> a. heart rate within acceptable range (state specific highest and lowest rate for each child)

In order to individualize this statement, the nurse needs to include the highest and lowest acceptable heart rate range for each child. The range will vary depending upon age and disease state. The expected outcome for a one-month-old infant with normal cardiac function would read:

> Child will have adequate cardiac output as evidenced by
>
> a. heart rate between 100 and 160 beats/minute

Possible Nursing Interventions: These are ways the nurse can assist the child and/or family to achieve the expected outcomes. Some of these interventions are *independent* nursing actions, while others are *collaborative* (as the nurse implements the physician's orders). For example, a nursing intervention to "elevate the head of the bed 30°" could be instituted on a child with increased intracranial pressure without a specific order from the physician. This would be an independent nursing intervention. A nursing intervention to "ensure antibiotic is administered on schedule" is dependent upon the physician's orders.

Evaluation for Charting: This is the final step in the nursing process. This section evaluates the expected outcomes and, to some extent, the identified nursing interventions. Statements made here direct the reader to answer questions or to describe or state results. For example, the reader may be directed to "describe breath sounds." This would be correlated with the expected outcome "child will have clear and equal breath sounds" and a nursing intervention such as "assess and record child's breath sounds every two hours and prn."

The evaluation statement may need to be changed frequently. For this reason the nurse may wish to include this part of the nursing process in the daily charting; if so, the nurse would note it on the nursing care plan under the evaluation column "See nurses' notes," and state date, time, and initials.

Related Nursing Diagnoses: These are nursing diagnoses that are most likely to be included in a nursing care plan for a child with the stated medical diagnosis. Many of these nursing diagnoses are either potential or actual nursing diagnoses; the nurse determines which. The related nursing diagnoses are in priority order for a child with the stated medical diagnosis. However, the needs and condition of the child will determine whether the nurse needs to reorder the priorities. All related nursing diagnoses are completely developed through the nursing process and can be found in the text; refer to the index for location.

A separate section is included on those nursing diagnoses that are unrelated to specific medical diagnoses. All such diagnoses have been included in the *Related Nursing Diagnoses*.

To use this book most efficiently, scan the table of contents for the applicable medical diagnosis. After finding it in the text, review the accompanying nursing care plan and related nursing diagnoses, and select the appropriate expected outcomes and nursing interventions. Write those on the nursing care plan, then implement them. Later, at intervals you designate when writing the care plan, evaluate the child's response to your nursing interventions and chart your findings.

With this Nursing Diagnosis Pocket Guide, **Neonatal and Pediatric Nursing Care Plans**, you will organize your nursing practice around nursing diagnoses, the professional level of practice.

Section I
Neonatal Care Plans

A. Care Plans for Common Medical Diagnoses Medical Diagnosis with Accompanying Primary Nursing Diagnosis

Medical Diagnosis **BRONCHOPULMONARY DYSPLASIA**

Primary Nursing Diagnosis **IMPAIRED GAS EXCHANGE**

Definition Alteration in the exchange of oxygen and carbon dioxide in the lungs and/or at the cellular level

Possibly Related to

Long-term ventilator therapy
Barotrauma from mechanical ventilation
High oxygen concentration
Alveolar rupture or pulmonary interstitial emphysema

Characteristics

Cyanosis
Retractions
Nasal flaring
Tachycardia
Diminished or unequal breath sounds
Abnormal blood gas values

Expected Outcomes

Infant will maintain adequate gas exchange as evidenced by

a. lack of
   —cyanosis
   —retractions
   —nasal flaring
b. heart rate within acceptable range of 100 to 160 beats/minute
c. respiratory rate within acceptable range of 30 to 60 breaths/minute
d. clear and equal breath sounds
e. arterial blood gas values within acceptable range (state specific highest and lowest values for each infant)

Possible Nursing Interventions

Assess and record

- signs/symptoms of impaired gas exchange (such as those listed under Characteristics) every 2 hours and prn
- breath sounds every 2 hours and prn
- arterial blood gas results as ordered; notify physician if results are out of the acceptable stated range
- infant's axillary temperature as ordered

Give oxygen in correct amount and route of delivery. State effectiveness of treatment.

Assess patency of endotracheal tube by listening to breath sounds every 15 minutes.

Suction endotracheal tube every 2 hours and prn.

Maintain sterile technique when suctioning.

Oxygenate infant prior to treatments (e.g., suctioning) as indicated.

Check ventilator settings (including CPAP) every 15 minutes. Record settings every 1 to 2 hours.

Change infant's position every 2 hours.

Ensure chest physiotherapy is being done effectively and gently on schedule.

Maintain a neutral thermal environment.

Evaluation for Charting

Did infant demonstrate any signs/symptoms of impaired gas exchange?

Describe breath sounds.

State highest and lowest respiratory and heart rates.

Describe amount and characteristics of secretions that resulted from suctioning the infant.

Was oxygenation prior to treatments effective in reducing hypoxia?

State highest and lowest arterial blood gas values, and state the on-going physiologic process.

Was infant's position changed every 2 hours?

Was chest physiotherapy effective in improving gas exchange?

Was a neutral thermal environment maintained?

State highest and lowest temperatures.

Did infant demonstrate adequate gas exchange?

Related Nursing Diagnoses

Ineffective breathing pattern related to

a. long-term ventilator therapy
b. high oxygen concentration

Ineffective airway clearance related to

a. endotracheal tube
b. increased secretions

Decreased cardiac output related to increased pulmonary vascular resistance

Ineffective family coping related to

a. long-term hospitalization of infant
b. financial difficulties of family

Medical Diagnosis

CONGESTIVE HEART FAILURE

Primary Nursing Diagnosis

DECREASED CARDIAC OUTPUT

Definition

A decrease in the amount of blood that leaves the left ventricle

Possibly Related to

Fluid volume overload
Increased pressure in the lungs
Increased flow to the lungs
Congenital heart defect
Noncardiovascular disease such as respiratory disease or anemia

Characteristics

Tachycardia
Tachypnea
Dyspnea
Rales
Cyanosis
Hepatosplenomegaly
Feeding difficulties
Fatigue
Weak or bounding peripheral pulses
Cough
Edema

Expected Outcomes

Infant will maintain an adequate cardiac output as evidenced by

a. heart rate within acceptable range of 100 to 160 beats/minute
b. respiratory rate within acceptable range of 30 to 60 breaths/minute
c. lack of cyanosis
d. strong and equal peripheral pulses bilaterally
e. clear and equal breath sounds

Infant will be free of signs/symptoms of congestive heart failure such as

a. dyspnea
b. hepatosplenomegaly
c. fatigue
d. feeding difficulty

Possible Nursing Interventions

Assess and record

- vital signs every 2 hours and prn
- breath sounds every 2 hours and prn
- murmurs every 2 hours and prn
- femoral, brachial, and pedal pulses every 2 hours and prn
- signs/symptoms of congestive heart failure every 2 hours and prn
- urine specific gravity every 8 hours
- percent of oxygen liter flow, route of oxygen delivery, and effectiveness of treatment

Maintain and record accurate intake and output.

Organize nursing care to allow for rest periods in order to decrease the workload on the heart.

Keep infant in semi-Fowler's position (e.g., infant seat)

Evaluation for Charting

State highest and lowest heart and respiratory rates.

Describe breath and heart sounds.

State presence and strength of peripheral pulses.

State presence and degree of any signs/symptoms of congestive heart failure.

State intake and output. Does the infant have fluid excess or fluid deficit?

State highest and lowest urine specific gravities.

State amount and route of oxygen delivery. Describe effectiveness of treatment.

Was infant kept in the semi-Fowler's position?

Related Nursing Diagnoses

Impaired gas exchange related to alteration in cardiac output

Fluid volume excess related to alteration in cardiac output

Alteration in nutrition: less than body requirements related to

a. dyspnea
b. tachypnea
c. fatigue

Ineffective family coping related to infant's life-threatening medical diagnosis

Medical Diagnosis

HYALINE MEMBRANE DISEASE/RESPIRATORY DISTRESS SYNDROME

Primary Nursing Diagnosis

IMPAIRED GAS EXCHANGE

Definition

Alteration in the exchange of oxygen and carbon dioxide in the lungs and/or at the cellular level

Possibly Related to

Decreased production of surfactant
Immature lung tissue

Characteristics

Tachypnea
Diminished or unequal breath sounds
Retractions (supracostal, intracostal, or subcostal)
Nasal flaring
Grunting
Cyanosis
Tachycardia
Abnormal blood gas values

Expected Outcomes

Infant will maintain adequate gas exchange as evidenced by

a. respiratory rate within acceptable range of 30 to 60 breaths/minute
b. clear and equal breath sounds
c. mild to no retractions
d. lack of
   —nasal flaring
   —expiratory grunt
   —cyanosis
e. heart rate within acceptable range of 100 to 160 beats/minute
f. arterial blood gas values within acceptable range (state specific highest and lowest values for each infant)

Possible Nursing Interventions

Assess and record

- breath sounds every 2 hours and prn
- signs/symptoms of impaired gas exchange (such as those listed under Characteristics) every 2 hours and prn

Give oxygen in correct amount and route of delivery. State effectiveness of treatment.

Assess patency of endotracheal tube by listening to breath sounds every 15 minutes.

Suction endotracheal tube every 2 hours.

Oxygenate infant prior to treatments (such as suctioning) as indicated.

Assess and record arterial blood gas results as ordered. Notify physician if results are out of the acceptable stated range.

Check ventilator settings (including CPAP) every 15 minutes. Record settings every 1 to 2 hours.

Change infant's position every 2 hours.

Ensure chest physiotherapy is being done effectively and gently on schedule.

Maintain a neutral thermal environment.

Assess and record infant's axillary temperature and Isolette or warmer temperature every 2 hours and prn.

Evaluation for Charting

Did infant demonstrate adequate gas exchange?

Did infant display any signs/symptoms of impaired gas exchange?

Describe breath sounds.

State highest and lowest respiratory and heart rates.

Was oxygenation prior to treatments effective in reducing hypoxia?

State highest and lowest arterial blood gas values, and state the on-going physiologic process.

Describe amount and characteristics of secretions that resulted from suctioning the infant.

Were the chest physiotherapy treatments effective in improving gas exchange?

Was infant's position changed every 2 hours?

State highest and lowest temperatures.

Was a neutral thermal environment maintained?

Related Nursing Diagnoses

Ineffective breathing pattern related to

a. long-term ventilator therapy
b. high oxygen concentration
c. impaired surfactant

Ineffective airway clearance related to increased secretions

Potential for infection related to

a. suctioning
b. endotracheal tube
c. immature immune system

Fluid volume deficit related to

a. insensible water loss from rapid respiratory rate
b. inability to tolerate fluids by mouth

Alteration in nutrition: less than body requirements related to inability to tolerate feedings by mouth resulting from respiratory distress

Decreased cardiac output related to impaired oxygenation

Ineffective family coping related to

a. illness of infant
b. financial difficulties of family
c. younger/older age of parents
d. single-parent situation
e. location of family home (e.g., out of town)
f. lack of support system for parents/family

Medical Diagnosis

HYPERBILIRUBINEMIA

Primary Nursing Diagnosis

ALTERATION IN LEVEL OF CONSCIOUSNESS*

Definition

Impaired state of awareness; can range from mild to complete impairment (coma)

Possibly Related to

Deposition of unconjugated bilirubin in the brain cells resulting from

- breakdown of red blood cells
- impaired excretion, overproduction, and/or deficient conjugation of bilirubin
- isoimmunization from blood-type or Rh incompatibility

Characteristics

Jaundice
Lethargy
Poor feeding
Edema
Ascites
Dark-colored urine
Clay-colored stools
Pruritus
Seizures
High-pitched cry

Expected Outcomes

Infant will be free of signs/symptoms of hyperbilirubinemia as evidenced by

a. lack of
—jaundice
—lethargy
—edema or ascites
—pruritus
—seizures

---

*Not NANDA approved at publication

b. total serum bilirubin level less than 1.5 mg/ml
c. ability to tolerate feedings
d. pale-yellow urine
e. yellow-brown stools
f. normal tone of cry

Possible Nursing Interventions

Assess and record

- infant's skin for color and signs of itching every shift
- signs of edema or ascites; measure abdominal girth if ordered and record results
- any neurologic changes in infant with vital signs every 2 hours
- results of arterial blood gases if ordered since acidosis causes increased levels of free unbound bilirubin and causes the albumin binding of bilirubin to weaken
- Dextrostix as ordered; hypoglycemia will cause the breakdown of fats to yield free fatty acids that displace bilirubin from albumin

Assess bilirubin levels when they are ordered. Notify physician if levels are increasing.

Keep infant unclothed under phototherapy lights with eyes covered. Remove infant (and eye pads) from lights for short periods to hold or have parents hold and comfort.

Keep accurate record of intake and output. Record characteristics of urine and stools. Anticipate increased fluid needs due to evaporative loss.

Prevent chilling of infant to avoid raising levels of free fatty acids that displace bilirubin from its albumin-binding sites.

Prepare infant and family for exchange transfusion if indicated. Explain procedure and rationale for doing procedure to the family. Follow hospital protocol for doing exchange transfusion. Monitor infant's vital signs continuously during exchange transfusion.

Evaluation for Charting

State infant's color.

State highest and lowest bilirubin levels.

Was phototherapy used? Was infant kept under lights unclothed with eye pads?

State any signs/symptoms of hyperbilirubinemia noted.

State intake and output and characteristics of urine and stools.

State neurologic status.

State highest and lowest temperatures.

State highest and lowest arterial pHs if ordered.

Was an exchange transfusion done? If so, describe infant's level of tolerance for procedure.

Related Nursing Diagnoses

Alteration in nutrition: less than body requirements related to poor sucking and lethargy

Alteration in level of consciousness related to the deposition of unconjugated bilirubin in brain cells

Potential for infection related to sepsis or intrauterine infection

Decreased cardiac output related to hemorrhage and polycythemia

Impaired skin integrity related to pruritus and drying of skin resulting from phototherapy

Fluid volume deficit related to evaporative loss and/or diarrhea resulting from phototherapy

Medical Diagnosis — # HYPOGLYCEMIA

Primary Nursing Diagnosis — ## ALTERATION IN NUTRITION: LESS THAN BODY REQUIREMENTS

Definition Insufficient amount of glucose in the blood

Possibly Related to

Limited ability to mobilize glycogen stores
Increased utilization of glucose due to physiologic stress

Characteristics

Jitteriness, Tremors
Apnea
Irregular respirations
Tachypnea
Lethargy
Irritability
Seizures
Poor feeding
High-pitched, weak cry
Hypothermia

Expected Outcomes

Infant will have an adequate blood glucose level as evidenced by

a. Dextrostix reading above 45 and below 160
b. serum glucose between 40 (30 in preterm infants) and 100 mg/dl
c. regular respiratory rate within acceptable range of 30 to 60 breaths/minute
d. lack of
   —jitteriness
   —tremors
   —seizures
   —lethargy
   —extreme irritability
e. no decrease in appetite

f. normal tone of cry
g. heart rate within acceptable range of 100 to 160 beats/minute
h. axillary temperature between 36.5° and 37.2° C

Possible Nursing Interventions

Assess and record Dextrostix and serum glucose levels as ordered. Notify physician if values are low.

Assess and record

- vital signs every 2 hours and prn
- signs/symptoms of hypoglycemia

Keep accurate record of intake and output including hourly record of IV fluids and IV site.

Evaluation for Charting

State highest and lowest Dextrostix and serum glucose levels.

State highest and lowest temperatures, respiratory and heart rates.

State intake and output. Describe any problems encountered with IV or IV site.

Describe any signs/symptoms of hypoglycemia noted.

Related Nursing Diagnoses

Alteration in level of consciousness related to lack of glucose to central nervous system

Impaired gas exchange related to increased oxygen consumption

Ineffective breathing pattern related to tachypnea and apnea

Decreased cardiac output related to poor cardiac contractility

Medical Diagnosis

HYPOTHERMIA

Primary Nursing Diagnosis

ALTERATION IN THERMOREGULATION*

Definition

Instability of the infant's body temperature

Possibly Related to

Large surface-to-weight ratio
Lack of subcutaneous fat
Limited shivering response

Characteristics

Decreased body temperature
Increased oxygen needs
Hypoglycemia
Decreased respirations
Bradycardia
Edema of the extremities
Decreased appetite
Restlessness
Agitation

Expected Outcomes

Infant will be free of signs/symptoms of altered thermoregulation as evidenced by

a. axillary temperature between 36.5° and 37.2° C
b. stable oxygen needs
c. serum glucose values between 45 and 100 mg/dl (or Dextrostix above 45)
d. respiratory rate within acceptable range of 30 to 60 breaths/minute
e. heart rate within acceptable range of 100 to 160 beats/minute
f. lack of
—edema

---

*Not NANDA approved at publication

—extreme restlessness or agitation

g. no decrease in appetite

Possible Nursing Interventions

Assess and record

- infant's vital signs every 2 hours and prn
- signs/symptoms of hypothermia

Ensure a neutral thermal environment is maintained. Note changes in ambient temperature, skin temperature, and heater output as related to axillary temperature.

Always use alarms and skin probes when using infant warmers and Isolettes.

Place plastic sheet or bubble bag over infants in open warmers when indicated.

Keep infant away from air drafts.

Keep Isolettes and open warmers away from windows or drafty areas. Prewarm any surface infant is to be placed on, such as x-ray plate.

Keep infant dry. Change as soon as possible after elimination.

Evaluation for Charting

State highest and lowest vital signs.

Describe any signs/symptoms of hypothermia noted.

Describe any successful methods used to help prevent hypothermia.

Was a neutral thermal environment maintained?

Were oxygen needs stable?

State highest and lowest glucose levels.

Related Nursing Diagnoses

Impaired gas exchange related to increased oxygen needs

Ineffective breathing pattern related to decreased respirations

Decreased cardiac output related to bradycardia

Alteration in nutrition: less than body requirements related to decreased appetite

Medical Diagnosis

INTRAVENTRICULAR HEMORRHAGE

(Usual sites are the lateral and third ventricles)

Primary Nursing Diagnosis

ALTERATION IN LEVEL OF CONSCIOUSNESS*

Definition

Impaired state of awareness; can range from mild to complete impairment (coma)

Possibly Related to

- Impaired gas exchange
- Venous congestion or increased cerebral venous pressure
- Arterial overperfusion
- Impaired autoregulation of the cerebral circulation
- Complication from use of volume expanders
- Increased intrapleural pressure
- Complication of a pneumothorax (from transmission of the positive pressure from the ventilator in the pleural space)
- Complication from use of hyperosmolar solutions (bicarbonate)
- Unknown etiology

Characteristics

- Ashen color
- Hypotonia
- Apnea
- Generalized or focal seizures
- Unresponsiveness
- Temperature instability
- Taut or bulging anterior fontanel
- Metabolic acidosis
- Increased head circumference

---

*Not NANDA approved at publication

Expected Outcomes

Infant will demonstrate a normal level of consciousness, and will be free of any signs/symptoms of intraventricular hemorrhage as evidenced by

a. lack of
   —cyanosis or ashen color
   —hypotonia
   —seizure activity
b. regular respiratory rate of 30 to 60 breaths/minute
c. stable temperature between 36.5° and 37.2° C
d. flat anterior fontanel
e. arterial blood gas values within acceptable range (state specific highest and lowest values for each infant)

Possible Nursing Interventions

Assess and record

- infant's color every 2 hours and prn
- neurologic signs, including movement and strength of extremities, every 2 hours and prn
- respiratory rate and temperature every 2 hours and prn
- condition of anterior fontanel every 2 hours and prn
- arterial blood gas results as ordered; notify physician if results are out of the acceptable stated range
- amount and route of oxygen delivery
- head circumference daily

Assess frequently for any signs of apnea. Record any apneic spells as they occur.

Maintain a neutral thermal environment.

Organize nursing care to minimize excessive handling of infant in order to help prevent hypoxia.

Maintain a safe environment for the infant in order to prevent any injury to the soft cranium. Consider using water-filled mattress.

Evaluation for Charting

Did infant demonstrate a normal level of consciousness?

Did infant display any signs/symptoms of intraventricular hemorrhage?

State highest and lowest respiratory rates and temperatures.

Was a neutral thermal environment maintained?

Describe condition of anterior fontanel.

State highest and lowest arterial blood gas values, and state the on-going physiologic process.

State amount, route, and effectiveness of oxygen delivery.

State measurement of head circumference and determine if it is an increase or decrease from the previous measurement.

Related Nursing Diagnoses

Impaired gas exchange related to

a. gestational age
b. immature lung tissue
c. increased intrapleural pressure

Decreased cardiac output related to

a. hypoxia
b. venous congestion
c. arterial overperfusion

Potential for injury related to soft cranium

Ineffective family coping related to

a. possibility of neurologically handicapped infant
b. increased length of hospital stay
c. potential for developmental delay

Medical Diagnosis — **MECONIUM ASPIRATION**

Primary Nursing Diagnosis — **INEFFECTIVE AIRWAY CLEARANCE**

Definition — Inability to adequately clear secretions from the airways

Possibly Related to — Attempt of infant to breathe in utero as a result of

- prolonged or difficult labor
- interference with the supply of oxygen via the placenta
- asphyxial episodes in utero that lead to extrauterine increase in pulmonary vascular resistance

Characteristics —
Tachypnea
Abnormal breath sounds (i.e., rales, rhonchi)
Cyanosis
Labored respirations (grunting and retractions)
Hypoxia
X-ray shows marked air trapping and hyperexpansion

Expected Outcomes — Infant will clear airway adequately as evidenced by

a. clear and equal breath sounds
b. respiratory rate within acceptable range of 30 to 60 breaths/minute
c. lack of cyanosis and labored respirations
d. arterial blood gas values within acceptable range (state specific highest and lowest values for each infant)
e. clear chest x-ray

f. white blood cell count within acceptable range of 5,000 to 21,000 mm^3

Possible Nursing Interventions

Assess and record

- breath sounds every 2 hours and prn
- signs/symptoms of ineffective airway clearance every 2 hours and prn
- amount and characteristics of any pulmonary secretions

Maintain sterile technique when deep suctioning.

Ensure oxygen is being delivered in the correct amount and route if ordered. Record percent of flow, route of delivery, and effectiveness of treatment.

Ensure that chest physiotherapy is being done effectively and gently on schedule.

Check and record results of chest x-ray and laboratory data when indicated.

Ensure antibiotics are administered on schedule. Assess for side effects such as rash or diarrhea.

Evaluation for Charting

Describe breath sounds.

State amount and route of oxygen delivery that was maintained. Describe effectiveness of therapy.

Did infant display any signs/symptoms of ineffective airway clearance as noted in Characteristics?

Describe amount and characteristics of any pulmonary secretions.

Were the chest physiotherapy treatments effective in loosening secretions?

State any laboratory results if appropriate.

State results of chest x-ray if appropriate.

Were antibiotics given on schedule? Describe any side effects noted.

Related Nursing Diagnoses

Ineffective breathing pattern related to ineffective airway clearance

Impaired gas exchange related to ineffective airway clearance

Fluid volume deficit related to

a. increased insensible water loss from rapid respirations
b. lethargy
c. fatigue

Alteration in nutrition: less than body requirements related to respiratory distress

Ineffective family coping related to illness of a newborn infant

Medical Diagnosis

NECROTIZING ENTEROCOLITIS

Primary Nursing Diagnosis

ALTERATION IN NUTRITION: LESS THAN BODY REQUIREMENTS

Definition

Insufficient nutrients to meet body needs

Possibly Related to

Decreased perfusion to the gastrointestinal tract
Hypoxia
Formula feedings
Hypertonic feedings
Polycythemia
Complication of umbilical artery catheterization
Anaerobic infection

Characteristics

Temperature instability
Abdominal distention
Inability to tolerate feedings
Faint or absent bowel sounds
Failure to gain weight
Erythema at umbilicus
Bile-stained, coffee-ground, or bloody vomitus
Bloody diarrhea
Hepatosplenomegaly
Slow capillary refill
Positive stool tests for blood and reducing sugars
Decreased blood platelets
Abdominal x-rays show dilated loops of intestine and gas bubbles in the wall of the intestine

Expected Outcomes

Infant will be free of signs/symptoms of nutritional deficit as evidenced by

a. temperature between 36.5° and 37.2° C

b. absence of abdominal distention; stable abdominal girth (measured just above umbilicus)
c. active bowel sounds
d. ability to retain and tolerate oral feedings
e. minimal (2 to 3 cc) to no residual prior to tube feeding
f. lack of
—vomiting
—diarrhea
—jaundice
—erythema around umbilicus
—hepatosplenomegaly
h. negative stool tests for occult blood and reducing sugars
i. platelet count between 100,000 and 300,000 mm^3
j. negative abdominal x-ray films for distended loops of intestine and visible gas bubbles in the walls of the intestine
k. weight gain of 10 to 20 grams/day

Possible Nursing Interventions

Assess and record

- for abdominal distention every shift; measure and record abdominal girth every day and prn
- bowel sounds every shift
- signs/symptoms of necrotizing enterocolitis (such as those described under Characteristics) every 2 hours and prn
- vital signs every 2 hours and prn
- capillary refill every 2 hours and prn
- daily weight on same scale without clothes

Keep accurate record of intake and output including gastric residual prior to tube feeding. Check stools for blood and reducing sugars when indicated.

Provide mouth care every shift if infant is npo.

Assess NG tube for position and patency every 2 hours. Connect it to low intermittent suction or gravity drainage (as ordered).

Assess area around umbilicus every 4 hours. Record and notify physician if any erythema or other abnormalities are present.

Assess infant's color every shift. Record any abnormalities.

Evaluation for Charting

Describe abdominal assessment.

State abdominal girth and indicate if it is an increase, decrease, or the same as the previous measurement.

State weight and indicate if it is an increase or decrease from the previous weight.

Describe any signs/symptoms of necrotizing enterocolitis.

State intake and output including gastric residual.

State results of blood or reducing-sugars tests on stools when indicated.

State highest and lowest vital signs.

Was NG tube patent and in place? Describe characteristics of any drainage.

Describe area around umbilicus.

Describe capillary refill.

Describe skin color.

Related Nursing Diagnoses

Decreased cardiac output related to

a. hypoxia

b. polycythemia
c. bleeding from the gastrointestinal tract

Fluid volume deficit related to

a. vomiting
b. diarrhea
c. bleeding from the gastrointestinal tract

Potential for infection related to

a. immature immune system
b. umbilical artery catheter

Ineffective family coping related to

a. increased length of hospital stay for infant
b. possibility of surgery for bowel resection

Medical Diagnosis

PATENT DUCTUS ARTERIOSUS

Primary Nursing Diagnosis

IMPAIRED GAS EXCHANGE

Definition

Alteration in the exchange of oxygen and carbon dioxide in the lungs and/or at the cellular level

Possibly Related to

Hypoxemia and poorly developed ductal muscle wall resulting in patent fetal circulatory opening between the pulmonary artery and the aorta

Characteristics

Tachypnea
Expiratory grunting
Intercostal retractions
Crackling rales
Murmur
Wide pulse pressure
Bounding peripheral pulses
Tachycardia
Hepatomegaly
Edema

Expected Outcomes

Infant will have adequate gas exchange and will be free of signs/symptoms of a patent fetal circulatory opening as evidenced by

a. respiratory rate within acceptable range of 30 to 60 breaths/minute
b. lack of
   —expiratory grunting
   —retractions
   —hepatomegaly
   —cardiac murmur
c. clear and equal breath sounds
d. pulse pressure within acceptable range of 20 to 50 mmHg

e. strong (nonbounding) and equal peripheral pulses
f. heart rate within acceptable range of 100 to 160 beats/minute
g. adequate urinary output of 1/2 to 1 cc/kg/hr

Possible Nursing Interventions

Ensure oxygen is being delivered in the correct amount and route (if ordered). Record percent of flow, route of delivery, and effectiveness of treatment.

Assess and record

- breath sounds with vital signs every 2 hours and prn
- signs/symptoms of respiratory distress (such as those listed under Characteristics) every 2 hours and prn
- vital signs, including blood pressure, every 2 hours and prn; note pulse pressure and peripheral pulses every 2 hours and prn
- position of liver every 8 hours and prn

Maintain a neutral thermal environment.

Administer indomethacin if ordered and assess for any side effects (e.g., edema, infection, impaired renal and hepatic function).

Keep accurate record of intake and output.

Evaluation for Charting

Describe breath sounds.

State amount and route of oxygen delivery that was maintained. Describe effectiveness.

Did infant display any signs/symptoms of respiratory distress?
State highest and lowest respiratory and heart rates and blood pressures.
Describe heart sounds.
Were peripheral pulses strong and equal?
Describe position of liver.
Describe any side effects of indomethacin noted.
Was a neutral thermal environment maintained?
State intake and output.

Related Nursing Diagnoses

Decreased cardiac output related to

a. cardiac defect
b. increased flow on the right side of the heart
c. increased workload on the right side of the heart

Fluid volume excess related to

a. cardiac defect
b. increased flow on the right side of the heart
c. increased workload on the right side of the heart
d. decreased blood flow to the kidneys

Alteration in nutrition: less than body requirements related to hypoxemia and decreased blood flow to the gastrointestinal tract

Ineffective family coping related to

a. defect of a major organ
b. increased time of hospital stay for infant

Medical Diagnosis

PERSISTENT FETAL CIRCULATION

Primary Nursing Diagnosis

IMPAIRED GAS EXCHANGE

Definition

Alteration in the exchange of oxygen and carbon dioxide in the lungs and/or at the cellular level

Possibly Related to

Airway obstruction from meconium aspiration
Hyperviscosity of the blood
Space-occupying lesion of the chest
Lung hypoplasia
Chronic intrauterine hypoxia
Maternal placental insufficiency
Prenatal pulmonary hypertension
Congenital heart disease
Interference with pulmonary vessel growth

Characteristics

Persistent cyanosis despite attempts to ventilate with oxygen
Tachypnea
Systolic murmur
Poor capillary perfusion
Seizures (if severely asphyxiated)
Unequal radial and umbilical artery blood gas values

Expected Outcomes

Infant will have adequate gas exchange as evidenced by

a. diminished cyanosis or lack of cyanosis
b. respiratory rate within acceptable range of 30 to 60 breaths/minute
c. lack of cardiac murmur
d. rapid capillary refill

e. equal radial and umbilical artery blood gas values
f. arterial blood gas values within acceptable range (state specific highest and lowest values for each infant)

Possible Nursing Interventions

Assess and record

- respiratory rate every 2 hours and prn
- any cardiac murmur every 2 hours and prn
- vital signs including blood pressure every 2 hours and prn
- arterial blood gas results as ordered; notify physician if results are out of the acceptable stated range

Ensure oxygen is being delivered in the correct amount and route. Record percent of flow and route of delivery. Assess for effectiveness of treatment.

Check setting on ventilator frequently. Record settings every 2 hours.

Suction endotracheal tube every 2 hours and prn. Use sterile technique when suctioning.

Assess patency of endotracheal tube by listening to breath sounds and checking the pressure setting on the ventilator every 15 to 30 minutes.

Maintain a neutral thermal environment.

Assess effects of vasodilators, smooth muscle relaxants (e.g., curare, Pavulon), and volume expanders (e.g., fresh frozen plasma) if ordered.

Evaluation for Charting

State highest and lowest respiratory rates.
State amount, route, and effectiveness of oxygen delivery.
State highest and lowest ventilatory settings.
Describe amount and characteristics of secretions that resulted from suctioning the infant.
Describe any problems encountered with patency of the endotracheal tube.
Did infant have a cardiac murmur?
Describe capillary refill.
State highest and lowest arterial blood gas values, and state the on-going physiologic process. Were radial and umbilical artery blood gas values unequal?
Was a neutral thermal environment maintained?
State if vasodilators, smooth muscle relaxants, and/or volume expanders were given. Describe their effectiveness.
State intake and output.
Was infant's position changed every 2 hours?

Related Nursing Diagnoses

Decreased cardiac output related to hypotension and/or shock
Alteration in level of consciousness related to hypoxia and acidosis
Alteration in nutrition: less than body requirements related to decreased blood flow to the gastrointestinal tract

Fluid volume excess related to hypoperfusion to the kidneys
Ineffective family coping related to life-threatening illness of infant

Medical Diagnosis

PNEUMONIA

Primary Nursing Diagnosis

INEFFECTIVE AIRWAY CLEARANCE

Definition

Inability to adequately clear secretions from the airways

Possibly Related to

An infection of the lungs resulting from

- pooling of secretions secondary to lack of adequate cough reflex
- immature immune response as a result of prematurity
- transplacental passage of microorganisms
- passage of microorganisms from infant's ascent through the birth canal
- nosocomial spread of organisms

Characteristics

Tachypnea
Cyanosis
Abnormal breath sounds (i.e., rales, crackles, rhonchi, wheezes)
Hypo- or hyperthermia
Apnea

Expected Outcomes

Infant will clear airway adequately as evidenced by

a. clear and equal breath sounds
b. lack of
 —cyanosis
 —apnea
c. respiratory rate within acceptable range of 30 to 60 breaths/minute
d. arterial blood gas values within acceptable range (state specific highest and lowest values for each infant)

e. temperature within acceptable range of 36.5° to 37.2° C
f. white blood cell count within acceptable range of 5,000 to 21,000 mm^3
g. clear chest x-ray

Possible Nursing Interventions

Ensure oxygen is being delivered in the correct amount and route if ordered. Record percent of liter flow, route of delivery, and effectiveness of treatment.

Assess and record

- breath sounds and vital signs every 2 hours and prn
- signs/symptoms of lung congestion every 2 hours and prn
- amount and characteristics of any pulmonary secretions
- infant's temperature every 2 hours and prn

Maintain sterile technique when deep suctioning.

Ensure chest physiotherapy is being done effectively and gently on schedule.

Maintain a neutral thermal environment.

Check and record results of chest x-ray and laboratory data (such as tracheal aspirate) when indicated.

Ensure antibiotics are administered on schedule. Assess for any side effects such as rash or diarrhea.

Evaluation for Charting

Describe breath sounds.

State amount and route of oxygen delivery that was maintained. Describe effectiveness.

Did infant display any signs/symptoms of lung congestion?

Were the chest physiotherapy treatments effective in loosening secretions?

State highest and lowest temperatures.

Was a neutral thermal environment maintained?

State any laboratory results if appropriate.

State results of chest x-ray if appropriate.

Were antibiotics given on schedule? Describe any side effects noted.

Related Nursing Diagnoses

Ineffective breathing pattern related to ineffective airway clearance

Impaired gas exchange related to ineffective airway clearance

Fluid volume deficit related to

a. increased insensible water loss from rapid respirations
b. lethargy
c. fatigue

Alteration in nutrition: less than body requirements related to respiratory distress

Alteration in comfort related to chest pain

Alteration in thermoregulation related to infection of the lungs

Ineffective family coping related to increased length of hospital stay for infant

Medical Diagnosis

PNEUMOTHORAX

Primary Nursing Diagnosis

IMPAIRED GAS EXCHANGE

Definition

Alteration in the exchange of oxygen and carbon dioxide in the lungs and/or at the cellular level

Possibly Related to

Collapsed lung (or collapsed portion of a lung) resulting from

- fetal distress
- difficult delivery
- meconium aspiration
- high ventilatory pressures

Characteristics

Grunting
Nasal flaring
Retractions
Cyanosis
Bradycardia
Diminished or unequal breath sounds
Unequal chest expansion
Abnormal arterial blood gas values

Expected Outcomes

Infant will maintain adequate gas exchange as evidenced by

a. lack of
  —grunting
  —nasal flaring
  —retractions
  —cyanosis
b. heart rate within acceptable range of 100 to 160 beats/minute
c. clear and equal breath sounds
d. equal chest expansion bilaterally
e. arterial blood gas values within acceptable range (state specific

highest and lowest values for each infant)

Possible Nursing Interventions

Assess and record

- signs/symptoms of impaired gas exchange (such as those listed under Characteristics) every 2 hours and prn
- breath sounds and vital signs every 2 hours and prn
- arterial blood gas results as ordered; notify physician if results are out of the acceptable stated range
- results of chest x-ray if appropriate
- percent of liter flow and route of oxygen delivery if appropriate; assess for effectiveness of treatment

Check pressure settings on ventilator and/or CPAP every 15 minutes. Record settings every 2 hours.

Prepare infant for any medical treatments such as surgical puncture or insertion of chest tube.

Explain any indicated procedures and rationale to the infant's family.

Maintain a neutral thermal environment.

Change infant's position every 2 hours.

Ensure chest physiotherapy is being done effectively and gently, on schedule.

Evaluation for Charting

Did infant demonstrate adequate gas exchange?

Did infant display any signs/symptoms of impaired gas exchange?

Describe breath sounds.

State highest and lowest arterial blood gas values, and state the on-going physiologic process.

State highest and lowest pressure settings on the ventilator and/or CPAP.

Describe infant's level of tolerance for any procedures that might have been done such as surgical puncture or chest tube insertion.

If a medical procedure was done, did the infant show any improvement in gas exchange following the procedure?

State results of chest x-ray if appropriate.

State amount and route of oxygen delivery that was maintained. Describe effectiveness.

State highest and lowest temperatures.

Was a neutral thermal environment maintained?

Was infant's position changed every 2 hours?

Was chest physiotherapy effective in improving gas exchange?

Related Nursing Diagnoses

Potential for infection related to

a. surgical puncture wound
b. insertion of chest tube

Fluid volume deficit related to inability to tolerate fluids by mouth resulting from respiratory distress

Ineffective family coping related to

a. illness of the infant
b. need for additional invasive procedures

Medical Diagnosis

PULMONARY INTERSTITIAL EMPHYSEMA

Primary Nursing Diagnosis

IMPAIRED GAS EXCHANGE

Definition

Alteration in the exchange of oxygen and carbon dioxide in the lungs and/or at the cellular level

Possibly Related to

Air leaks from the base of the alveoli into the interstitial perivascular space

Positive airway pressure supplied by a ventilator and/or CPAP

Characteristics

Tachypnea
Retractions
Cyanosis
Irritability
Restlessness
Respiratory acidosis
Hypotension

Expected Outcomes

Infant will maintain adequate gas exchange as evidenced by

a. respiratory rate within acceptable range of 30 to 60 breaths/minute
b. lack of
 —retractions
 —cyanosis
 —extreme irritability
 —extreme restlessness
c. arterial blood gas values within acceptable range (state specific highest and lowest values for each infant)
d. blood pressure within acceptable range of 64 to 96 mmHg systolic and 30 to 62 mmHg diastolic

Possible Nursing Interventions

Assess and record

- breath sounds every 2 hours and prn
- signs/symptoms of impaired gas exchange (such as those listed under Characteristics) every 2 hours and prn
- arterial blood gas results as ordered; notify physician if results are out of the acceptable stated range
- percent of liter flow and route of oxygen delivery every 2 hours; assess effectiveness of treatment
- infant's temperature every 2 hours and prn

Check pressure settings on the ventilator and/or CPAP frequently (every 15 to 30 minutes). Record settings every 2 hours.

Prepare infant for any medical treatments such as surgical puncture or insertion of chest tube.

Explain any procedures and rationale to the infant's family.

Note and record results of chest x-ray if appropriate.

Maintain a neutral thermal environment.

Change infant's position every 2 hours.

Evaluation for Charting

State highest and lowest respiratory rates.

Did infant display any signs/symptoms of impaired gas exchange?

Did infant demonstrate adequate gas exchange?

State highest and lowest arterial blood gas values, and state the on-going physiologic process.

State highest and lowest blood pressures.

State highest and lowest pressures on the ventilator and/or CPAP.

Describe infant's level of tolerance for any procedures that were done (e.g., surgical puncture or chest tube drainage).

Did the infant show any improvement in gas exchange after the procedure?

State results of chest x-ray if appropriate.

State amount and route of oxygen delivery maintained. Describe effectiveness of treatment.

State highest and lowest temperatures.

Was a neutral thermal environment maintained?

Was infant's position changed every 2 hours?

Related Nursing Diagnoses

Ineffective breathing pattern related to air leaks from the base of the alveoli into the interstitial perivascular space

Potential for infection related to

a. surgical puncture wound
b. insertion of chest tube drainage

Fluid volume deficit related to

a. insensible water loss from rapid respiratory rate
b. inability to tolerate fluids by mouth

Alteration in nutrition: less than body requirements related to inability to tolerate feedings by mouth secondary to respiratory distress

Ineffective family coping related to

a. illness of the infant
b. need for additional invasive procedures

Medical Diagnosis **SEPSIS**

Primary Nursing Diagnosis **POTENTIAL FOR INFECTION***

Definition A condition in which the body is invaded by microorganisms

Possibly Related to

Immature immune system
Intrauterine infection
Nosocomial source
Unknown etiology

Characteristics

Temperature instability
Tachypnea
Periodic breathing
Apnea
Tachycardia
Lethargy
Feeding intolerance
Petechiae

Expected Outcomes

Infant will be free of infection as evidenced by

a. temperature between 36.5° and 37.2° C
b. regular respiratory rate between 30 and 60 breaths/minute
c. heart rate between 100 and 160 beats/minute
d. lack of
 —extreme lethargy
 —petechiae
e. white blood cell count within normal limits of 5,000 to 21,000 mm^3

---

*Not NANDA approved at publication

Possible Nursing Interventions

Assess and record

- axillary temperature every 2 hours and prn
- signs/symptoms of infection every 2 hours and prn

Maintain a neutral thermal environment.

Ensure antibiotics are given on schedule. Assess for any side effects such as rash or diarrhea.

Keep accurate record of intake and output.

Assess IV site every hour for signs/symptoms of infection or infiltration

Use sterile technique when doing specific treatments such as suctioning and changing IV tubing.

Maintain good handwashing technique, especially between patients.

Assess parents'/visitors' knowledge of handwashing technique; correct as needed.

Check results of cultures such as tracheal aspirate and blood cultures.

Check and record results of CBC.

Evaluation for Charting

State highest and lowest body temperatures, respiratory and heart rates.

Was a neutral thermal environment maintained?

Describe any signs/symptoms of infection that were noted.

Were antibiotics given on schedule? Describe any side effects noted.

State intake and output.

Describe IV site.

Did parents/visitors demonstrate correct handwashing technique?

State results of any cultures and/or CBC if available.

Related Nursing Diagnoses

Ineffective breathing pattern related to tachypnea and/or periodic breathing

Fluid volume deficit related to

a. fever
b. decreased appetite
c. side effects of antibiotics

Decreased cardiac output related to tachycardia

Ineffective family coping related to

a. illness of infant
b. present illness resulting in prolonged hospital stay

Medical Diagnosis: TRANSIENT TACHYPNEA OF THE NEWBORN

Primary Nursing Diagnosis: INEFFECTIVE BREATHING PATTERN

Definition

A breathing pattern that results in insufficient oxygen to meet the cellular requirements of the body

Possibly Related to

Delay in absorption of fetal lung fluids

Characteristics

Tachypnea (usually in excess of 80 breaths/minute)
Cyanosis in room air
Air trapping seen on chest x-ray
Barrel chest
Minimal retractions

Expected Outcomes

Infant will maintain an effective breathing pattern as evidenced by

a. respiratory rate within acceptable range of 30 to 60 breaths/minute
b. lack of
   —retractions
   —cyanosis with less than 50% oxygen requirement
   —air trapping on chest x-ray
c. disappearance of barrel chest
d. clear and equal breath sounds

Possible Nursing Interventions

Assess and record

- vital signs and breath sounds every 2 hours and prn
- signs/symptoms of impaired breathing pattern every 2 hours and prn
- percent of liter flow and route of oxygen delivery; assess for effectiveness of treatment

Maintain a neutral thermal environment.

Change infant's position every 2 hours.

Evaluation for Charting

State highest and lowest respiratory rates.

Describe breath sounds.

Did infant display any signs/symptoms of ineffective breathing pattern?

State amount and route of oxygen delivery maintained. Describe effectiveness of treatment.

Was a neutral thermal environment maintained?

State highest and lowest temperatures.

Was infant's position changed every 2 hours?

Related Nursing Diagnoses

Impaired gas exchange related to retained fetal lung fluid

Fluid volume deficit related to

a. insensible water loss from rapid respirations
b. inability to tolerate fluids by mouth

Alteration in nutrition: less than body requirements related to inability to tolerate feedings by mouth resulting from the rapid respiratory rate

Ineffective family coping related to the unexpected illness of the infant (usually occurs in term or slightly preterm infants)

Neonatal Care Plans
B. Additional Nursing Diagnoses

Nursing Diagnosis **ANTICIPATORY GRIEVING: PARENTAL/FAMILY**

Definition Feelings (or individual is at risk for feelings) of deep sadness and distress

Possibly Related to

Critical state of infant's illness
Separation from infant
Physical defects of infant
Infant death

Characteristics

Verbal expression of grief by parents/family
Sadness
Crying, screaming
Inability to carry on with activities of daily living at an optimal level
Need for repeated explanations and reassurance
Passivity

Expected Outcomes

Parents/family will grieve appropriately as evidenced by

a. crying quietly
b. talking and asking questions about the infant
c. seeking help and advice appropriately
d. performing activities of daily living at an adequate level

Possible Nursing Interventions

Allow parents/family to grieve in their own way, and give them support.

Encourage parents/family to spend time with their infant if it seems to help their grieving process.

If possible, have the same nurse(s) care for infant from day to day in order to provide consistent feedback for parents.

Allow parents/family to participate in the care of the infant when possible. Examples: rubdowns with Vitamin E cream, dressing changes, naming baby, baptism, changing diaper, etc.

Allow parents/family to spend time alone at their infant's bedside if possible.

Spend time with the parents/family when possible.

Keep parents/family up to date on the condition of their infant.

When possible, have family make tapes of their voices that can be played for infant.

Evaluation for Charting

Did parents/family verbalize any feeling of grief?

Describe any signs/symptoms of grief displayed by parents/family.

Were parents/family able to carry on with activities of daily living?

Describe any successful measures used to help parents/family cope with their grief.

Nursing Diagnosis: FLUID VOLUME EXCESS

Definition

Increased (or infant is at risk for increased) circulating fluid volume in the body

Possibly Related to

Immature kidneys
Excess fluid intake
Excess sodium intake
Complication from nephrotoxic antibiotic therapy
Cardiac defect

Characteristics

Edema
Ascites
Bulging fontanels
Excessive weight gain
Restlessness or lethargy
Irritability
Moist rales
Dyspnea
Weak, rapid, irregular heart rate
Increased blood pressure
Low specific gravity

Expected Outcomes

Infant will regain normal fluid balance as evidenced by

a. lack of edema or ascites
b. flat fontanels
c. steady, predictable weight gain of 10 to 30 grams/day
d. lack of
   —restlessness
   —lethargy
   —extreme irritability
e. regular respiratory rate of 30 to 60 breaths/minute
f. clear and equal breath sounds

g. regular and strong heart rate within acceptable range of 100 to 160 beats/minute
h. blood pressure within acceptable range of 64 to 96 mmHg systolic and 30 to 62 mmHg diastolic
i. specific gravity between 1.008 and 1.020

Possible Nursing Interventions

Keep accurate record of intake and output.

Assess and record for any signs/symptoms of fluid overload every 2 hours and prn. Notify physician if any signs/symptoms are observed.

Weigh infant nude on the same scale at approximately the same time each day.

Assess and record infant's breath sounds, respiratory and heart rates, and blood pressure every 2 hours and prn.

Assess and record specific gravity every void.

Evaluation for Charting

State intake and output.

Describe any signs/symptoms of fluid overload observed.

State infant's weight and determine if it is an increase or decrease from previous weight.

State highest and lowest respiratory and heart rates and blood pressures.

Describe infant's breath sounds.

State highest and lowest specific gravities.

Nursing Diagnosis — IMPAIRMENT OF SKIN INTEGRITY

Definition

Interruption (or the individual is at risk for interruption) in integrity of the skin

Possibly Related to

Fragile tissue
Decreased amount of brown fat

Characteristics

Discoloration of skin (reddened area)
Pressure over bony prominences
Open or draining areas on skin
Change in elasticity of skin

Expected Outcomes

Infant will be free of signs/symptoms of impaired skin integrity as evidenced by

a. no reddened or discolored areas of skin
b. lack of
   —constant pressure over bony prominences
   —open or draining areas
c. no change in elasticity of skin

Possible Nursing Interventions

Handle infant gently.
Encourage others (e.g., parents, visitors, x-ray personnel) to handle infant gently.
Bathe daily with water (soap when indicated).
Use baby lotion to lubricate skin when indicated.
Decrease use of tape and electrodes when possible.
Carefully remove tape and electrodes when necessary.
Assess and record skin condition every shift.
Turn infant every 2 hours.

Consider using sheepskin blankets, water beds, egg crates, etc.

Change diaper as soon as possible after elimination.

Treat any breakdown areas or potential areas as soon as they are discovered by keeping area clean and dry, exposing area to air if indicated, and applying medication or ointment, if ordered.

Evaluation for Charting

Describe any potential or actual areas of skin breakdown.

Was infant's position changed every 2 hours?

Nursing Diagnosis INEFFECTIVE FAMILY COPING

Definition Inability of family members to effectively manage problems and concerns

Possibly Related to

Illness of infant
Financial difficulties
Young/old age of parents
Single-parent situation
Location of family home (e.g., out of town)
Lack of support system

Characteristics

Inability to express fears and concerns
Inability to ask for and accept outside help
Unwillingness to participate in infant's care
Failure to understand repeated explanations and rationale for treatments and procedures
Inability to meet own basic needs such as eating and rest
Inappropriate anger towards staff

Expected Outcomes

Family will be able to cope appropriately as evidenced by

a. being able to express fears and concerns to members of the health care team
b. knowing when it is appropriate to seek outside help
c. accepting outside help when it is warranted
d. participating in care of their infant when indicated
e. verbalizing understanding of rationale for necessary treatments and procedures

f. caring for own basic needs such as getting appropriate rest and eating meals

Possible Nursing Interventions

Communicate with parents/family concerning their infant's condition at least once/shift and prn as the infant's condition demands. This may require telephoning the parents when they are not able to come to the hospital.

Encourage family to express their fears and concerns.

Identify and record any past or usual successful coping strategies used by family.

Assist family in seeking outside help when indicated.

Allow and encourage family to participate in the care of the infant when possible.

Explain procedures and treatments to the parents/family.

Give reasons and rationale for doing procedures and treatments.

Assist and encourage family to meet own basic needs such as eating and resting appropriately.

Evaluation for Charting

Describe any fears or concerns expressed by the family.

Was family willing to accept outside help if indicated?

Did family participate in the care of the infant when indicated?

Was family able to understand the necessity and rationale for treatments and procedures?

Were family members able to meet their own basic needs?
State any successful measures used to help family's coping ability.

Nursing Diagnosis **KNOWLEDGE DEFICIT, PARENTAL/FAMILY**

Definition Lack of information by parents/family concerning the care of their infant

Possibly Related to

Sensory overload (too much to learn all at once)

Fear of emotional involvement with an infant that may die

Cognitive or cultural-language limitations

Guilt or anger at having delivered a premature infant

Characteristics

Verbalization by parents/family indicating lack of knowledge

Relating incorrect information to members of the health care team

Inability to correctly repeat and comprehend information taught to parents/family

Inability to correctly demonstrate skills that have been previously taught

Inappropriate or hostile behavior towards staff

Expected Outcomes

Parents/family will have an adequate knowledge base concerning the care of their infant as evidenced by

a. being able to correctly state information they have been taught
b. being able to correctly demonstrate skills they have been taught
c. lack of inappropriate or hostile attitude towards the staff

Possible Nursing Interventions

Listen to the parents' and/or family members' concerns and fears.

Give parents/family correct information and literature (when available) on the care and treatment of their infant.

Dispel any incorrect information that the parents and/or family members may have.

Assist and observe parents/family in performing skills they have been taught regarding the care of their infant. Record their ability to perform skills.

Be nonjudgmental of parents and/or family members concerning their previous actions.

Assign a primary nurse as usual spokesperson to family.

Evaluation for Charting

Did parents/family verbalize a knowledge deficit?

Were parents/family able to correctly state information they have been taught?

Were parents/family able to perform skills previously taught? If so, describe ability of parents/family to perform the skills.

Describe any inappropriate or hostile attitude of parents/family.

Section II: Pediatric Care Plans

A. Care Plans for Common Medical Diagnoses

Medical Diagnosis

ASTHMA OR REACTIVE AIRWAY DISEASE

Primary Nursing Diagnosis

IMPAIRED GAS EXCHANGE

Definition

Alteration in the exchange of oxygen and carbon dioxide in the lungs and/or at the cellular level

Possibly Related to

Spasms of the smooth muscle of the bronchi and bronchioles
Accumulation of tenacious secretions
Edema of the mucous membranes of the airways
Allergies
Infection

Characteristics

Wheezing
Tachypnea
Decreased breath sounds
Retractions
Nasal flaring
Cough
Anxiety
Fatigue

Expected Outcomes

Child will have adequate gas exchange as evidenced by

a. clear and equal breath sounds bilaterally
b. respiratory rate within acceptable range (state specific highest and lowest rates for each child)
c. lack of
—wheezing
—nasal flaring
d. absence of respiratory retractions
e. decreased or absent cough
f. decreased anxiety

g. decreased fatigue
h. arterial blood gas results within acceptable range if indicated (state specific range for each child)

Possible Nursing Interventions

Assess and record every 2 hours and prn

- breath sounds
- signs/symptoms of impaired gas exchange (such as those listed under Characteristics)

Assess effectiveness of

- oxygen in correct amount and specified route of delivery as ordered; record percent of liter flow and route of delivery
- bronchodilators and steroids as ordered

Be sure chest physiotherapy is done at appropriate times. Chart effectiveness of the treatments.

Keep head of bed elevated at a 30° to 45° angle.

Evaluation for Charting

Describe breath sounds.

State highest and lowest range of respiratory rate.

Describe any signs/symptoms of impaired gas exchange noted.

State whether oxygen was given, amount and route of delivery. Describe effectiveness.

Describe effectiveness of chest physiotherapy treatments if appropriate.

Was head of bed kept elevated?

Related Nursing Diagnoses

Fluid volume deficit related to

a. respiratory distress
b. increased insensible water loss from rapid respiratory rate

Fear, child's related to

a. respiratory distress
b. hospitalization

Ineffective family coping related to

a. repeated hospitalization of child
b. respiratory distress of child

Medical Diagnosis

BRONCHIOLITIS

Primary Nursing Diagnosis

INEFFECTIVE BREATHING PATTERN

Definition

A breathing pattern that results in insufficient oxygen to meet the cellular requirements of the body

Possibly Related to

A viral inflammatory infection of the lower airways

Characteristics

Tachypnea
Retractions
Nasal flaring
Rales
Grunting
Fever
Cough
Wheezing
Cyanosis

Expected Outcomes

Child will have an effective breathing pattern as evidenced by

a. clear and equal breath sounds bilaterally
b. respiratory rate within acceptable range (state specific highest and lowest rates for each child)

Decrease in or lack of

a. retractions
b. nasal flaring
c. grunting
d. cough
e. cyanosis
f. fever

Possible Nursing Interventions

Assess and record every 2 hours and prn

- breath sounds
- signs/symptoms of ineffective breathing pattern (such as those listed under Characteristics)

Administer humidified oxygen (if ordered) in correct amount and route of delivery. Record percent of liter flow and route of delivery. Assess for effectiveness of therapy.

Ensure chest physiotherapy is done as ordered. Assess for effectiveness of the treatments.

Suction child prn if child is unable to clear airway.

Evaluation for Charting

Describe breath sounds.

State highest and lowest respiratory rates.

Describe any signs/symptoms of ineffective breathing pattern noted.

State whether oxygen was given and give amount and route of delivery. Describe effectiveness.

Describe effectiveness of chest physiotherapy.

Did child need suctioning? If so, describe characteristics of secretions.

Related Nursing Diagnoses

Fluid volume deficit related to

a. respiratory distress
b. decreased fluid intake
c. increased insensible water loss from rapid respirations

Alteration in nutrition: less than body requirements related to

a. respiratory distress
b. refusal of solid foods
c. lethargy

Sleep pattern disturbance related to

a. respiratory distress
b. unfamiliar surroundings
c. possible hypoxia

Ineffective family coping related to

a. hospitalization of child
b. stress of seeing child with respiratory distress

Medical Diagnosis

BURNS

Primary Nursing Diagnosis

FLUID VOLUME DEFICIT

Definition

A decrease in the amount of circulating fluid volume

Possibly Related to

Vascular to interstitial fluid shift
Hot liquid burn (scalds)
Open flame burn
Electrical source burn
Caustic or chemical agent burn

Characteristics

Edema
Decreased urinary output
Elevated urine specific gravity
Elevated serum creatinine
Elevated serum BUN
Burn wound characteristics

- first degree—erythematous, painful; blanches on pressure and refills
- second degree—blistered, erythema, very painful; blanches on pressure and refills
- third degree—skin appears white or charred, little pain; does not blanch and refill on pressure

Expected Outcomes

Child will have an adequate fluid volume as evidenced by

a. adequate urinary output (state specific highest and lowest outputs for each child)
b. receiving ordered amount of fluid therapy (state exact amount/hour that is ordered)

c. urine specific gravity between 1.008 and 1.020
d. serum creatinine level between 0.3 and 1.1 mg/dl
e. serum BUN level between 5 and 20 md/dl

Possible Nursing Interventions

Keep accurate record of intake and output.

Check and record flow of IV fluids and condition of IV site every hour.

Assess and record

- urinary output every hour (or as ordered)
- urine specific gravity every 4 hours
- laboratory values as indicated
- condition of burn wound once/shift and prn

Apply dressings to burn wound as ordered.

Evaluation for Charting

State intake and output.

Describe condition of IV site.

State highest and lowest urine specific gravities.

State current laboratory values. If any were abnormal, state action taken.

Describe burn wound.

Related Nursing Diagnoses

Electrolyte imbalance: sodium and potassium related to tissue damage and the burn injury

Potential for injury, infection related to impaired skin integrity and decreased resistance

Alteration in comfort: pain related to burn injury

Alteration in nutrition: less than body requirements related to high metabolic requirements and catabolism

Impairment of skin integrity related to burn injury

Ineffective family coping related to

a. possible parental guilt
b. severity of burn injury
c. pain child is experiencing
d. painful treatments and procedures child needs
e. long-term and/or future hospitalizations

Disturbance in self-concept: body image related to future scar tissue

Impaired physical mobility related to future scarring and contractures

Medical Diagnosis

CARDIAC CATHETERIZATION, POSTPROCEDURE

Primary Nursing Diagnosis

DECREASED CARDIAC OUTPUT

Definition

A decrease in the amount of blood that leaves the left ventricle

Possibly Related to

Dysrhythmias
Cardiac perforation
Hemorrhage
Arterial or venous obstruction

Characteristics

Dysrhythmias, bradycardia, or tachycardia
Hypotension
External or internal bleeding
Absence of pulse in involved extremity distal to entry site
Coolness, cyanosis, or blanching of involved extremity distal to entry site

Expected Outcomes

Child will have adequate cardiac output as evidenced by

a. normal sinus rhythm
b. heart rate within acceptable range (state specific highest and lowest rates for each child)
c. blood pressure within acceptable range (state specific highest and lowest pressures for each child)
d. adequate pulse in involved extremity
e. lack of coolness, cyanosis, or blanching of involved extremity

Possible Nursing Interventions

Assess and record

- vital signs including blood pressure every 15 minutes until stable,

then every 1 hour for 8 hours, then every 4 hours
- color, skin temperature
- signs/symptoms of hemorrhage (refer back to Characteristics) distal to entry site of the involved extremity; use Doppler if necessary
- condition of dressing site with vital signs

Keep the involved extremity straight for 8 hours.

Give diet as ordered after child is fully awake.

Give antipyretics as ordered for temperature above 38.3° C. Check temperature 1 hour after administration of medication for effectiveness.

Ensure Lanoxin elixir is administered on schedule. Assess for side effects such as nausea and bradycardia. Check heart rate prior to administering medication. Hold medication and check with physician before giving if heart rate is below 100 in infants.

Evaluation for Charting

State highest and lowest vital signs.

State condition of involved extremity.

Describe condition of dressing site.

Was involved extremity kept straight?

Was diet tolerated?

If antipyretics were necessary, state effectiveness.

Related Nursing Diagnoses

Potential for infection related to invasive procedure

Ineffective family coping related to outcome of procedure

Knowledge deficit, parental/family related to medical diagnosis confirmed by cardiac catheterization

Sleep pattern disturbance related to sedation used prior to and during procedure

Medical Diagnosis

CARDIOVASCULAR SURGERY, POSTOPERATIVE

Primary Nursing Diagnosis

DECREASED CARDIAC OUTPUT

Definition

A decrease in the amount of blood that leaves the left ventricle

Possibly Related to

Surgical complications such as

- thrombus
- ineffective circulation
- interference with electrical conduction
- hemorrhage

Dysrhythmias
Tachycardia or bradycardia
Decreased oxygenation

Characteristics

Tachycardia
Bradycardia
Dysrhythmias
Unequal, decreased, or absent peripheral pulses
Hemodynamic monitoring values outside the acceptable range
Slow capillary refill

Expected Outcomes

Child will maintain adequate cardiac output as evidenced by

a. heart rate within acceptable range (state specific highest and lowest rates for each child)
b. strong and equal peripheral pulses
c. blood pressure within acceptable range (state specific highest and lowest pressures for each child)

d. CVP within acceptable range (state specific highest and lowest values for each child)
e. pulmonary artery pressure value within acceptable range (state specific highest and lowest values for each child)
f. left atrial pressure value within acceptable range (state specific highest and lowest values for each child)
g. rapid capillary refill

Possible Nursing Interventions

Assess and record the following every hour and prn, reporting any changes to the physician

- vital signs, including blood pressure
- CVP reading
- left atrial pressure reading
- pulmonary artery pressure reading

Assess and record

- peripheral pulses (note if they are strong and equal)
- capillary refill

Compare vital signs with electronic monitoring devices.

Keep accurate record of intake and output.

Assess and record condition of dressing and/or incision site every shift and prn.

Use sterile technique when changing any of the central lines.

Maintain identification and integrity of pacer wires if present.

Evaluation for Charting

State highest and lowest values for each of the following

a. vital signs
b. CVP
c. left atrial pressure
d. pulmonary artery pressure

Were peripheral pulses strong and equal?
Describe capillary refill.
State intake and output.
Describe condition of dressing and incision site.

Related Nursing Diagnoses

Impaired gas exchange related to

a. surgical complications such as thrombus, ineffective circulation, or hemorrhage
b. decreased cardiac output
c. endotracheal intubation
d. chest tubes

Alteration in comfort, pain related to

a. surgical procedure
b. fear
c. anxiety

Potential for infection related to

a. surgical procedure
b. intubation
c. invasive monitoring

Ineffective family coping related to

a. child's surgery
b. child's hospitalization
c. fear of child dying
d. lack of support system
e. expense of procedure

Medical Diagnosis

CONGESTIVE HEART FAILURE

Primary Nursing Diagnosis

DECREASED CARDIAC OUTPUT

Definition

A decrease in the amount of blood that leaves the left ventricle

Possibly Related to

Fluid volume overload
Increased pressure in the lungs
Increased flow of blood to the lungs
Congenital heart defect
Acquired heart defect
Noncardiovascular disease such as respiratory disease or anemia

Characteristics

Tachycardia
Tachypnea, Dyspnea
Rales
Cyanosis
Hepatosplenomegaly
Feeding difficulties
Decline from the growth curve
Fatigue
Weak peripheral pulses
Edema (peripheral, periorbital, sacral)
Distended neck veins in older children
Diaphoresis
Weight gain
Cough
Cardiomegaly

Expected Outcomes

Child will maintain an adequate cardiac output as evidenced by

a. heart rate within acceptable range (state specific highest and lowest rates for each child)
b. respiratory rate within acceptable range (state specific highest and lowest rates for each child)

c. clear and equal breath sounds bilaterally
d. lack of
   —cyanosis
   —hepatosplenomegaly
   —feeding difficulty
   —fatigue
   —edema and excessive weight gain
   —cough
e. steady progress on the growth curve
f. strong and equal peripheral pulses bilaterally

Possible Nursing Interventions

Assess and record every 2 hours and prn

- apical heart rate
- breath sounds
- signs/symptoms of inadequate cardiac output (such as those listed under Characteristics)

Organize nursing care in order to allow child uninterrupted rest periods.

Administer cardiac drugs as ordered on schedule. Assess and record apical heart rate for 1 full minute prior to giving digoxin. Do not give medication if heart rate is below 100 beats/minute in child or as orders indicate.

Ensure diuretics are administered on schedule. Assess for any side effects such as dehydration and hypokalemia.

Elevate head of bed 10° to 30°.

Weigh daily at same time on same scale.

Evaluation for Charting

State highest and lowest range of child's heart and respiratory rates.

Describe breath sounds.

Describe any signs/symptoms of inadequate cardiac output noted.
State intake and output.
Were cardiac drugs and diuretics given on schedule? Describe any side effects noted.
Record weight. Was the weight an increase or decrease since the previous recorded weight?

Related Nursing Diagnoses

Impaired gas exchange related to

a. increased pressure in the lungs
b. increased flow of blood to the lungs
c. congenital heart defect
d. inadequate cardiac output

Fluid volume excess related to inadequate cardiac output

Alteration in nutrition: less than body requirements related to

a. decreased energy level
b. feeding difficulty
c. unknown etiology

Ineffective family coping related to

a. hospitalization of child
b. illness involving major body organ
c. added stress of chronic illness on family system

Medical Diagnosis

CYSTIC FIBROSIS

Primary Nursing Diagnosis

INEFFECTIVE AIRWAY CLEARANCE

Definition Inability to clear secretions from the airway

Possibly Related to

Excessive mucus
Bacterial infection

Characteristics

Diminished breath sounds
Cough
Tachypnea
Dyspnea
Wheezes, diffuse rales, and rhonchi
Frequent respiratory infections
Barrel-chest deformity
Cyanosis
Clubbing
Failure to gain weight
Malabsorption
Voracious appetite
Frequent foul-smelling stools
Hypernatremic "sweat" (skin tastes salty)

Expected Outcomes

Child will have adequate airway clearance as evidenced by

a. clear and equal breath sounds bilaterally
b. respiratory rate within normal limits (state specific highest and lowest rates for each child)
c. lack of cyanosis

Possible Nursing Interventions

Assess and record

- breath sounds and any signs/symptoms of respiratory distress (such as those listed under Characteristics) every 2 hours and prn

- amount and characteristics of secretions
- results of chest x-ray and CBC when indicated

Ensure that chest physiotherapy treatments are done every 2 hours while awake. Encourage child to cough during and after treatments.

Encourage child to spit out secretions in a tissue and dispose of tissue in waste container.

Ensure antibiotics are administered on schedule. Assess for side effects such as rash or diarrhea.

Encourage fluid intake in order to help liquify secretions.

Evaluation for Charting

Describe breath sounds.

State highest and lowest respiratory rates.

Describe any signs/symptoms of respiratory distress noted.

Indicate whether chest physiotherapy was done. Describe how child tolerated procedure, breath sounds before and after the treatment.

Describe secretions.

State whether antibiotics were given on schedule. Describe any side effects noted.

State results of chest x-ray and CBC when indicated.

Related Nursing Diagnoses

Impaired gas exchange related to excessive mucus

Alteration in nutrition: less than body requirements related to malabsorption

Ineffective family coping related to

a. long-term illness
b. fatal disease
c. financial considerations

Potential for infection related to invasion of the respiratory tract by bacterial organism

Guilt, parental/family related to the genetic nature of the disease

Decreased cardiac output related to increased pressure in the lungs resulting from hypoxia and hypercapnia secondary to thick secretions

Alteration in patterns of urinary elimination, retention related to side effects of antibiotic therapy

Medical Diagnosis

DIABETES MELLITUS, INSULIN-DEPENDENT (JUVENILE ONSET, TYPE I)

Primary Nursing Diagnosis

ALTERATION IN METABOLIC FUNCTION*

Definition

Imbalance in the body of the utilization of specific nutrients

Possibly Related to

Insufficient production of insulin

Characteristics

Hyperglycemia
Glycosuria
Polyuria
Polydipsia
Polyphagia
Weight loss
Abdominal or leg cramps
Emotional disturbances
Coma

Expected Outcomes

Child will have adequate metabolic functioning as evidenced by

a. stable blood sugar level between 60 and 180 mg/dl
b. lack of
 —glycosuria
 —signs/symptoms of hyperglycemia (e.g., weakness, increased thirst, frequent urination, dehydration, nausea and vomiting, abdominal pain, acetone breath, and rapid deep respirations)
 —weight loss

---

*Not NANDA approved at publication

Possible Nursing Interventions

Assess and record

- blood glucose levels as ordered
- signs/symptoms of hyperglycemia (such as those listed under Expected Outcomes) every 2 hours and prn
- signs/symptoms of hypoglycemia (e.g., mood change, irritability, shaky feeling, headache, hunger, impaired vision) every 2 hours and prn

Keep accurate record of intake and output.

Weigh child daily.

Allow child/family (depends on age of child) to do Chemstrips and/or urine testing as ordered. Assess and record technique observed.

Evaluation for Charting

State highest and lowest blood glucose levels.

Describe child's/family's technique.

Describe any signs/symptoms of hyperglycemia noted and action taken.

Describe any signs/symptoms of hypoglycemia noted and action taken. State intake and output.

State weight. Determine if it is an increase or decrease from the previous weight.

Related Nursing Diagnoses

Fluid volume deficit related to

a. polyuria
b. dehydration
c. vomiting
d. hyperglycemia resulting in osmotic diuresis

Knowledge deficit, parental/family related to disease state

Ineffective family coping related to

a. diagnosis of long-term illness
b. parental guilt from hereditary nature of the disease
c. uncertain prognosis for adulthood

Medical Diagnosis: DIABETIC KETOACIDOSIS

Primary Nursing Diagnosis: ALTERATION IN METABOLIC FUNCTION*

Definition
Imbalance in the body of the utilization of specific nutrients

Possibly Related to
Unstable blood glucose levels
Insufficient production of insulin
Increased insulin requirements resulting from infection, illness, or stress

Characteristics
Unstable blood glucose levels
Glycosuria
Acetone in urine
Weakness
Nausea and vomiting
Abdominal pain
Dehydration
Electrolyte imbalance
Acidosis
Coma

Expected Outcomes
Child will have adequate metabolic function as evidenced by

a. stable blood glucose level between 60 and 180 mg/dl
b. lack of
 —glycosuria/ketonuria
 —signs/symptoms of hyperglycemia (e.g., weakness, increased thirst, frequent urination, dehydration, nausea and vomiting, abdominal pain, acetone breath, and rapid deep respirations)

---

*Not NANDA approved at publication

—signs/symptoms of hypoglycemia (e.g., mood change, irritability, shaky feeling, headache, hunger, impaired vision)

Possible Nursing Interventions

Assess and record

- blood glucose levels every 2 hours and prn
- insulin drip every hour along with the condition of the IV site
- signs/symptoms of hyperglycemia or hypoglycemia (such as those listed under Expected Outcomes) every 2 hours and prn

Keep accurate record of intake and output.

Place child on cardiac monitor while receiving IV insulin. Notify physician of any abnormalities observed.

Evaluation for Charting

State highest and lowest blood glucose levels.

State highest and lowest Chemstrip and urine testing results.

State any signs/symptoms of hyperglycemia or hypoglycemia noted.

State intake and output.

Describe condition of IV site; give rate and amount of insulin drip.

Describe any abnormalities noted on the cardiac monitor.

Related Nursing Diagnoses

Fluid volume deficit related to

a. osmotic diuresis resulting from hyperglycemia
b. vomiting

Alteration in electrolyte balance: sodium and potassium related to

a. dehydration
b. vomiting

Alteration in nutrition: less than body requirements related to

a. decreased appetite
b. unstable blood glucose levels

Ineffective family coping related to

a. long-term illness and prognosis
b. need for continual monitoring of blood glucose, urine glucose, urine acetone, and diet on a daily basis

Medical Diagnosis

EPIGLOTTITIS

Primary Nursing Diagnosis

IMPAIRED GAS EXCHANGE

Definition

Alteration in the exchange of oxygen and carbon dioxide in the lungs and/or at the cellular level

Possibly Related to

An upper airway bacterial infection of the epiglottis that can cause total airway obstruction

Characteristics

Abrupt onset
Red, sore, inflamed throat
Difficulty or inability to swallow
Drooling of saliva
Muffled voice
Fever
Sits upright, refuses to lie down, head craned forward
Diminished breath sounds bilaterally
Substernal and suprasternal retractions
Tachypnea
Inspiratory stridor
Cyanosis
Anxious and frightened expression
Increased white blood cell count
Large, cherry-red, edematous epiglottis

Expected Outcomes

Child will have adequate gas exchange as evidenced by

a. patent airway
b. clear and equal breath sounds
c. respiratory rate within acceptable range (state specific highest and lowest rates for each child)
d. ability to swallow
e. lack of

—retractions
—inspiratory stridor
—cyanosis
—edema and discoloration of epiglottis

Possible Nursing Interventions

Assess and record

- breath sounds every 2 hours and prn
- signs/symptoms of impaired gas exchange or airway obstruction (such as those listed under Characteristics) every 2 hours and prn

Prior to intubation

- keep head of bed elevated at a 45° angle
- assess constantly for any signs/symptoms of increasing airway obstruction; record as indicated
- keep the following equipment at the bedside
  —endotracheal and tracheostomy tubes
  —oxygen equipment
  —suction equipment

After intubation

- suction, using sterile technique, every 2 hours and prn
- administer oxygen in the amount ordered; record percent of liter flow and route of delivery every 2 hours; assess for effectiveness of therapy

Allow and encourage family members to stay if it helps to decrease the child's anxiety.

Ensure antibiotics are administered on schedule. Assess for side effects such as rash or diarrhea.

Evaluation for Charting

Describe breath sounds.

State highest and lowest respiratory rates.

Describe any signs/symptoms of impaired gas exchange or airway obstruction noted.

Was child intubated? If so, state how often child was suctioned and describe characteristics of the secretions.

State amount and route of oxygen delivery. Describe effectiveness.

Did family members stay with the child and did it help to decrease the child's anxiety?

Were antibiotics administered on schedule? Describe any side effects noted.

Related Nursing Diagnoses

Fluid volume deficit related to

a. respiratory difficulty
b. sore throat
c. refusal to swallow
d. insensible water loss
   —from rapid respirations
   —due to increased temperature

Alteration in thermoregulation related to the bacterial infection in the upper respiratory tract as well as in the blood stream (septicemia) Fear, child's related to

a. respiratory difficulty
b. unfamiliar surroundings
c. forced contact with strangers
d. treatments and procedures

e. restraints

Ineffective family coping related to

a. hospitalization of child
b. life-threatening nature of illness
c. degree of respiratory distress child is experiencing
d. suddenness of onset of the illness

Medical Diagnosis

FAILURE TO THRIVE

Primary Nursing Diagnosis

ALTERATION IN NUTRITION: LESS THAN BODY REQUIREMENTS

Definition

Insufficient nutrients to meet body needs

Possibly Related to

Malabsorption
Loose stools
Decreased food intake
Possible problem with parent/child relationship
Congenital anomaly or other physical condition
Neglect
Possible parental knowledge deficit

Characteristics

Vomiting
Diarrhea
Lethargy
Apathy
Dehydration
Decline from growth curve
Developmental delay

Expected Outcomes

Child will be adequately nourished as evidenced by

a. lack of
   —vomiting
   —diarrhea
   —apathy and lethargy
b. steady weight gain (state how much would be reasonable for each child)
c. adequate caloric intake (state minimum number of calories needed for each child)

Possible Nursing Interventions

Keep accurate record of intake and output.

Weigh child daily at same time on same scale without clothes.

Feed child on schedule; record amount accurately.

Assist, observe, and record parental feeding technique (when appropriate).

Provide role modeling and education for feeding skills, infant care, and nurturing in a nonthreatening and nonjudgmental manner.

Evaluation for Charting

State intake and output.

State weight and determine if it is an increase or decrease from previous weight.

Describe child's eating behavior and any successful measures used that helped the child to eat.

Describe parent/child interaction and parent feeding technique.

Related Nursing Diagnoses

Fluid volume deficit related to

a. decreased fluid intake by mouth
b. loose stools

Ineffective family coping related to

a. diagnosis of failure to thrive in which no organic cause can be found
b. young age of parents
c. guilt over diagnosis
d. fear to bond with child because of a congenital anomaly

Developmental delay related to

a. nutritional deficit
b. parental knowledge deficit
c. lack of stimulation
d. repeated or long-term hospitalization

Medical Diagnosis

GASTROENTERITIS (DIARRHEA AND DEHYDRATION)

Primary Nursing Diagnosis

FLUID VOLUME DEFICIT

Definition

A decrease in the amount of circulating fluid volume

Possibly Related to

An infection: systemic (e.g., from a virus, bacteria, or parasite) or local (e.g., otitis media or a urinary tract infection)
Food or drug intolerance such as milk allergy
Inflammatory bowel disease such as ulcerative colitis
Malabsorption such as in cystic fibrosis
Psychogenic factors

Characteristics

Loose, watery stools (can be yellow or green and may contain mucus, blood, pus, or sugar)
Vomiting
Abdominal cramping
Abdominal distention
Hyperactive bowel sounds
Weight loss
Sunken fontanel
Sunken eyeballs
Poor skin turgor
Decreased urinary output

Expected Outcomes

Child will regain adequate fluid volume level as evidenced by

a. lack of
—diarrhea
—mucus, blood, pus, or sugar in the stool

—vomiting
—abdominal cramping and distention

b. adequate amount of IV and oral fluids (state exact amount of intake needed for each child)
c. normal activity of bowel sounds
d. regaining weight lost during illness
e. flat fontanel
f. normal orbital contour
g. rapid skin recoil
h. adequate urinary output (state specific highest and lowest outputs for each child)
i. urine specific gravity between 1.008 and 1.020

Possible Nursing Interventions

Keep accurate record of intake and output. Weigh diapers for urine and stool output (note frequency, color, odor, consistency, reducing substance). Measure vomitus.

Assess and record

- IV fluids and condition of IV site every hour
- bowel sounds every shift and prn
- signs/symptoms of fluid volume deficit (e.g., sunken fontanel or eyeballs, poor skin turgor) every 2 hours and prn

Weigh child daily on the same scale at the same time without clothes.

Give mouth care every 4 hours and prn.

Check and record urine specific gravity every void or as directed.

Report any of the following to the physician

- frequent stooling (more than 3 times/shift)
- large vomitus
- IV fluids infiltrated (not running)

Evaluation for Charting

State intake and output.
State condition of IV site.
Describe stools.
State weight and if it is an increase or decrease from the previous weight.
Describe status of fontanel, eyeballs, and skin turgor.
State highest and lowest urine specific gravities.
Was child adequately hydrated?

Related Nursing Diagnoses

Alteration in electrolyte balance: sodium and potassium related to diarrhea and vomiting.
Alteration in nutrition: less than body requirements related to vomiting and diarrhea
Decreased cardiac output related to poor perfusion secondary to dehydration
Impairment of skin integrity in the perineal area related to frequent and irritating stools
Ineffective family coping related to

a. hospitalization of child
b. unknown etiology

Medical Diagnosis

GLOMERULONEPHRITIS, ACUTE

Primary Nursing Diagnosis

FLUID VOLUME EXCESS

Definition

An increase in the amount of circulating fluid volume

Possibly Related to

Post-streptococcal infection
Antigen-antibody reaction
Pathologic changes in the glomeruli

Characteristics

Headache
Abdominal pain
Fever
Hematuria (Coke-colored urine)
Oliguria
Edema—especially periorbital (also scrotal)
Hypertension

Expected Outcomes

Child will regain fluid balance as evidenced by

a. adequate urinary output (state specific highest and lowest outputs for each child)
b. clear, pale-yellow urine
c. receiving only the ordered amount of fluid intake (state exact amount allowed for each child)
d. lack of
—edema
—headache
e. blood pressure within normal limits (state specific highest and lowest pressures for each child)
f. rapid weight gain

Possible Nursing Interventions

Keep accurate record of intake and output. Be sure child does not exceed maximum intake ordered. Document characteristics of urinary output.

Assess and record .

- signs/symptoms of fluid volume overload (such as those listed under Characteristics) every 2 hours and prn
- amount and location of edema once/shift
- blood pressure every 2 hours and prn

Weigh child daily on the same scale at the same time of day.

Evaluation for Charting

State intake and output.

Describe characteristics of urinary output.

Describe any signs/symptoms of fluid overload noted.

Describe amount and location of edema present.

State highest and lowest blood pressures.

State child's weight and determine if it is an increase or decrease from the previous weight.

Related Nursing Diagnoses

Alteration in level of consciousness

a. possible complication of hypertensive encephalopathy
b. electrolyte imbalance

Decreased cardiac output related to

a. hypertension
b. fluid volume overload

Alteration in nutrition: less than body requirements related to sodium and protein restriction

Alteration in tissue perfusion related to circulatory congestion

Alteration in patterns of urinary elimination, retention related to altered glomerular function

Disturbance in self-concept: body image related to edema

Ineffective family coping related to hospitalization of child

Medical Diagnosis

HIRSCHSPRUNG'S DISEASE, PREOPERATIVE

Primary Nursing Diagnosis

FLUID VOLUME DEFICIT

Definition

A decrease in the amount of circulating fluid volume

Possibly Related to

Poor feeding
Vomiting
Absence or scarcity of parasympathetic ganglion cells in some part of the lower bowel

Characteristics

Feeding problems
Dehydration, Weight loss
Vomiting (vomitus may include bile or fecal material)
Hypoproteinemia
Constipation
Passage of ribbon-like, foul-smelling stools
Overflow diarrhea
Visible peristalsis
Abdominal distention

Expected Outcomes

Child will be adequately hydrated as evidenced by

a. adequate fluid intake, IV or oral (state exact amount needed for each child)
b. adequate urinary output (state specific highest and lowest outputs for each child)
c. moist mucous membranes
d. flat fontanel
e. urine specific gravity below 1.020
f. rapid skin recoil

Possible Nursing Interventions

Keep accurate record of intake and output.

Assess and record

- IV fluid intake and condition of IV site every hour
- signs/symptoms of dehydration (such as those listed under Characteristics) every 2 hours and prn
- urine specific gravity once/shift

Evaluation for Charting

State intake and output.

Describe condition of IV site and any problems encountered with IV fluids.

Describe any signs/symptoms of dehydration noted.

State highest and lowest specific gravities.

Was child adequately hydrated?

Related Nursing Diagnoses

Alteration in nutrition: less than body requirements related to

a. poor feeding
b. vomiting

Alteration in bowel elimination: constipation related to absence or scarcity of parasympathetic ganglion cells in some part of the lower bowel

Alteration in comfort: pain related to

a. constipation
b. hunger

Ineffective family coping related to

a. hospitalization of child
b. impending surgery for colostomy
c. long-term prognosis

Medical Diagnosis

HYDROCEPHALUS

Primary Nursing Diagnosis

ALTERATION IN LEVEL OF CONSCIOUSNESS*

Definition

Reduced or impaired state of awareness; can range from mild to complete impairment (coma)

Possibly Related to

Increased intracranial pressure resulting from an increased amount of cerebrospinal fluid in the cerebrum as a consequence of increased production, decreased absorption, or obstruction

Characteristics

Vomiting
Poor feeding
Headache
Lethargy or irritability
Full or bulging fontanels
Increasing head circumference
Vision disturbance
Bulging eyes with "sunset sign"
Change in level of consciousness
High-pitched cry
Seizures
Pupillary changes

Expected Outcomes

Child will maintain an appropriate level of consciousness as evidenced by

a. lack of
 —headache
 —seizures
 —"sunset" sign
 —vomiting
b. being alert when awake
c. flat fontanels
d. stable head circumference

---

*Not NANDA approved at publication

e. pupils that are equal and react to light
f. normal-pitched cry

Possible Nursing Interventions

Assess and record

- neuro vital signs (e.g., changes in level of consciousness, orientation to time and place; pupillary changes; equal movement of extremities) with regular vital signs every 2 hours and prn
- signs/symptoms of increased intracranial pressure (see those listed under Characteristics) every 2 hours and prn
- age-related signs/symptoms of decreasing level of consciousness every 2 hours and prn (see Characteristics)

Measure and record head circumference.
Keep head in midline position.
Elevate head of bed 30°.
Keep accurate record of intake and output (overhydration can cause an increase in intracranial pressure).
Organize nursing care so patient can have uninterrupted rest periods to aid in decreasing intracranial pressure.

Evaluation for Charting

State results of neuro vital signs.
State any signs/symptoms of increasing intracranial pressure or of decreasing level of consciousness.
State head circumference and whether it is an increase or decrease since the previous measurement.

Was head of bed maintained at 30°, with head in midline position?
State intake and output.

Related Nursing Diagnoses

Impairment of skin integrity related to

a. thin and fragile skin of the head
b. pressure and weight of the head
c. inability of child to move head

Alteration in comfort: pain related to headache
Alteration in nutrition: less than body requirements related to increased intracranial pressure that can result in anorexia and vomiting
Fluid volume deficit related to increased intracranial pressure that can result in anorexia and vomiting
Ineffective family coping related to

a. seriousness of illness
b. underlying cause of illness
c. child's hospitalization
d. possibility of brain damage to child
e. possibility of long-term developmental problems of child
f. child's physical appearance

Medical Diagnosis

LARYNGOTRACHEOBRONCHITIS (CROUP)

Primary Nursing Diagnosis

INEFFECTIVE BREATHING PATTERN

Definition

A breathing pattern that results in insufficient oxygen to meet the cellular requirements of the body

Possibly Related to

A viral infection of the larynx, trachea, and bronchi

Characteristics

Tachypnea
Hoarseness
Brassy cough
Inspiratory stridor
Diminished breath sounds bilaterally
Substernal and suprasternal retractions
Fever
Irritability and restlessness
Pallor or cyanosis

Expected Outcomes

Child will have an effective breathing pattern as evidenced by

a. clear and equal breath sounds bilaterally
b. respiratory rate within acceptable range (state specific highest and lowest rates for each child)
c. lack of
 —signs/symptoms of increasing airway obstruction (e.g., stridor at rest, increasing restlessness or lethargy, retractions, cyanosis)
 —hoarseness and brassy cough

Possible Nursing Interventions

Assess and record every 2 hours and prn

- breath sounds with vital signs
- signs/symptoms of ineffective breathing pattern and increasing airway obstruction (such as those listed under Characteristics)

Administer cool mist by ordered route of delivery.

Assess effects of

- nebulized bronchodilators if ordered
- oxygen; be aware that over 40% oxygen may mask symptoms of increasing respiratory distress; arterial blood gases may be needed

Deep suction ONLY if it is specifically ordered. Suctioning may induce laryngospasms and cause further airway obstruction.

Evaluation for Charting

Describe breath sounds.

State highest and lowest respiratory rates.

Describe any signs/symptoms of ineffective breathing pattern or increasing airway obstruction noted.

State whether cool mist was administered and state the route of delivery.

If bronchodilators were given, state effectiveness.

Chart whether or not oxygen was given and state amount and route of delivery. State effectiveness of treatment.

Was suctioning needed? If so, describe any problems encountered during suctioning and state characteristics of secretions and response of patient.

Related Nursing Diagnoses

Fluid volume deficit related to

a. respiratory difficulty
b. sore throat
c. increased insensible water loss from rapid respirations

Fear, child's related to

a. respiratory distress
b. unfamiliar surroundings
c. forced contact with strangers
d. treatments and procedures
e. restraints

Ineffective family coping related to

a. hospitalization of child
b. respiratory distress of child

Medical Diagnosis

LEUKEMIA, ACUTE LYMPHOCYTIC

Primary Nursing Diagnosis

POTENTIAL FOR INFECTION*

Definition

Inability of the child's bone marrow to produce the right kind and/or amount of blood cells to protect against infection

Possibly Related to

Overproduction of atypical white blood cells
Decreased number of functional white blood cells
Bone-marrow suppression

Characteristics

Anemia
Thrombocytopenia
Neutropenia
Pallor
Increased bruising
Petechiae
Fatigue
Fever
Anorexia
Heptosplenomegaly
Bone and joint pain

Expected Outcomes

Child will have no signs/symptoms of infection.
Child will have normal level of blood-forming products as evidenced by

a. hematocrit within normal range (state specific highest and lowest hematocrit for each child)
b. hemoglobin within normal range (state specific highest and lowest hemoglobin for each child)

---

*Not NANDA approved at publication

c. platelet count between 150,000 and 450,000 mm^3
d. white blood cell count within normal range (state specific highest and lowest count for each child)
e. lack of pallor
f. disappearance of petechial rash

Possible Nursing Interventions

Monitor child for signs/symptoms of infection (e.g., fever, malaise).

Keep accurate intake and output.

Give blood products as ordered. Assess, record and report any signs/symptoms of transfusion reactions (e.g., chills, fever, headache, flank pain, urticaria, flushing, chest pain, difficulty breathing, irregular heart rate, apprehension).

Assess and record laboratory values as indicated.

Assess and record child's color and appearance of petechial rash.

Evaluation for Charting

State child's vital signs. State child's activity level and report of well-being.

State intake and output.

State type and amount of any blood products given, pre- and post-transfusion blood-work values. Describe any signs/symptoms of transfusion reaction.

Indicate if hematocrit, hemoglobin, platelets, and white blood cell values are increased or decreased from previous results.

Describe child's color and presence/absence of petechial rash.

Related Nursing Diagnoses

Ineffective family coping related to

a. serious illness of child
b. necessity of long-term therapy
c. necessary treatments and procedures
d. financial concerns
e. uncertain prognosis

Alteration in nutrition: less than body requirements related to side effects of chemotherapy drugs

Decreased cardiac output related to

a. anemia
b. decreased platelets

Disturbance in self-concept: body image related to

a. alopecia from chemotherapy
b. edema from steroid therapy

Alteration in comfort: pain related to

a. infiltration of leukemic cells into normal body tissue
b. diagnostic and treatment procedures (e.g., IVs, lumbar punctures)

Medical Diagnosis MENINGITIS

Primary Nursing Diagnosis ALTERATION IN LEVEL OF CONSCIOUSNESS*

Definition Reduced or impaired state of awareness; can range from mild to complete impairment (coma)

Possibly Related to An inflammation of the spinal cord, meninges, and the brain (state whether it is bacterial, viral, etc.)

Characteristics
Fever
Headache
Irritability
Lethargy
Vomiting
Poor feeding
Bulging fontanel
Nuchal rigidity
Change in level of consciousness
High-pitched cry
Pupillary changes
Positive Kernig and Brudzinski signs
Seizures
Apnea
Increase in head circumference

Expected Outcomes Child will maintain an appropriate level of consciousness as evidenced by

a. recognition of family members (if appropriate for age)
b. lack of lethargy
c. being alert when awake

Child will be free of signs/symptoms of increased intracranial pressure leading

---

*Not NANDA approved at publication

to a decrease in level of consciousness as evidenced by

a. no complaints of headache
b. lack of
   —extreme irritability
   —vomiting
   —seizures
   —apnea
   —increase in head circumference
c. flat, nonbulging fontanel
d. supple neck
e. normal-pitched cry
f. pupils that are equal and react to light
g. negative Kernig and Brudzinski signs

Possible Nursing Interventions

Assess and record

- neuro vital signs and regular vital signs at least every 2 hours and prn
- signs/symptoms of increased intracranial pressure every 2 hours and prn
- signs/symptoms of decreasing level of consciousness (such as those listed under Characteristics) every 2 hours and prn

Measure and record head circumference daily.

Elevate head of bed 30°.

Keep accurate record of intake and output (overhydration can cause an increase in intracranial pressure).

Organize nursing care so child can have uninterrupted rest periods to aid in decreasing intracranial pressure.

Ensure anticonvulsants are administered on schedule. Assess for side effects such as drowsiness, fatigue, and gastrointestinal upset.

Evaluation for Charting

State results of neuro vital signs.
State any signs/symptoms of increased intracranial pressure or any signs/symptoms of decreasing level of consciousness.
State head circumference and whether the value is an increase or decrease since the previous measurement.
Was head of bed maintained at 30°?
State intake and output.
Were anticonvulsants given on schedule? Describe any side effects noted.

Related Nursing Diagnoses

Alteration in thermoregulation related to the infection of the spinal cord, meninges, and brain

Alteration in comfort, pain related to

a. headache
b. neck pain
c. earache
d. fever

Ineffective family coping related to hospitalization of child with a serious illness

Potential developmental delay related to

a. possible increased intracranial pressure resulting in brain damage
b. infarcts
c. abscesses

Medical Diagnosis

OSTEOMYELITIS

Primary Nursing Diagnosis

POTENTIAL FOR INFECTION*

Definition

Invasion of the body by pathogenic organisms

Possibly Related to

Inflammation of the bone resulting from a hematogenous source, secondary to a wound or fracture

Characteristics

Fever
Pain in the affected extremity
Refusal to bear weight
Decreased range of motion
Localized tenderness
Localized warmth and redness
Localized swelling

Expected Outcomes

Child will be free of signs/symptoms of infection as evidenced by

a. body temperature between 36.5° and 37.2° C
b. lack of pain, tenderness, swelling, redness, and warmth to the affected extremity
c. white blood cell count within normal limits (state specific highest and lowest counts for each child)

Possible Nursing Interventions

Assess and record

- temperature with vital signs every 2 hours and prn
- signs/symptoms of infection (such as those listed under Characteristics) at least once/shift

---

*Not NANDA approved at publication

Administer antipyretic drugs as ordered.

Ensure antibiotics are administered on schedule. Assess for any side effects such as diarrhea or rash.

Handle affected limb gently.

Administer analgesics as ordered.

Evaluation for Charting

State highest and lowest temperatures.

Describe any signs/symptoms of infection noted.

If antipyretics were administered, state effectiveness.

Were antibiotics administered on schedule? Describe any side effects noted.

If analgesics were administered, state effectiveness.

Related Nursing Diagnoses

Alteration in comfort: pain related to inflammation of affected area

Impaired physical mobility related to inflammation of affected area and imposed immobility

Ineffective family coping related to

a. hospitalization of child
b. weeks of needed therapy
c. potential for long-term physical deformity

Medical Diagnosis

PNEUMONIA

Primary Nursing Diagnosis

IMPAIRED GAS EXCHANGE

Definition

Alteration in the exchange of oxygen and carbon dioxide in the lungs and/or at the cellular level

Possibly Related to

Infection of the lungs (state whether it is bacterial, viral, mycoplasma, etc.)

Characteristics

Tachypnea
Retractions
Rales, rhonchi
Change in respiratory secretions
Diminished breath sounds bilaterally
Cough
Fever
Chest pain
Abdominal pain
Cyanosis

Expected Outcomes

Child will have adequate gas exchange and will be free of signs/symptoms of a lung infection as evidenced by

a. clear and equal breath sounds bilaterally
b. respiratory rate within acceptable range (state specific highest and lowest rates for each child)
c. lack of
  —nasal flaring and retractions
  —cough
  —chest or abdominal pain
  —cyanosis
d. minimal clear secretions
e. temperature between 36.5° and 37.2° C
f. clear chest x-ray

Possible Nursing Interventions

Assess and record every 2 hours and prn

- breath sounds
- signs/symptoms of impaired gas exchange (such as those listed under Characteristics)
- signs/symptoms of lung infection

Ensure antibiotics are administered on schedule. Assess for any side effects such as rash or diarrhea.

Administer oxygen and humidified mist if ordered. Record route of delivery and percent of liter flow every 8 hours and prn. Assess effectiveness of therapy.

Ensure chest physiotherapy is done before meals if ordered.

Position child with head elevated when possible.

Evaluation for Charting

Describe breath sounds.

State highest and lowest respiratory rates and temperatures.

Describe signs/symptoms of impaired gas exchange or lung infection noted.

State amount and route of oxygen delivery. Describe effectiveness.

Were antibiotics given on schedule? Describe any side effects noted.

Describe effectiveness of chest physiotherapy if indicated.

Was child maintained in the head-elevated position?

Related Nursing Diagnoses

Fluid volume deficit related to

a. loss of desire to drink
b. anorexia

c. increased insensible water loss from rapid respirations
d. lethargy
e. fatigue

Alteration in nutrition: less than body requirements related to

a. respiratory distress
b. loss of appetite
c. anorexia
d. fever leading to increased caloric requirements

Alteration in thermoregulation related to the lung infection

Alteration in comfort, pain related to

a. chest pain
b. headache
c. cough
d. abdominal pain

Medical Diagnosis
PYLORIC STENOSIS, PREOPERATIVE

Primary Nursing Diagnosis
ALTERATION IN NUTRITION: LESS THAN BODY REQUIREMENTS

Definition
Insufficient nutrients to meet body needs

Possibly Related to
Thickening of the circular muscle of the pylorus

Characteristics
Projectile vomiting
Lack of bile in vomitus
Visible peristaltic waves
Palpable pyloric mass, "olive"
Dehydration

Expected Outcomes
Infant will be adequately nourished as evidenced by

a. lack of
   —vomiting
   —weight loss
b. absorbing adequate number of calories (state specific number needed for each infant)

Possible Nursing Interventions
Keep accurate record of intake and output. Record characteristics of vomitus and its relationship to feedings.
Give small frequent feedings slowly.
Bubble infant before and frequently during feedings.
Place infant in high-Fowler's position after feedings.
Organize care in order to decrease disturbing and handling infant after feedings.
Weigh daily on same scale at same time without clothes.

Evaluation for Charting

State intake and output.

Describe characteristics of vomitus and its relationship to feedings and infant behavior.

Was infant able to tolerate feedings? State any successful measures used that helped infant retain feedings.

State weight and determine if it is an increase or decrease from previous weight.

Related Nursing Diagnoses

Fluid volume deficit related to

a. vomiting
b. dehydration

Alteration in electrolyte balance: sodium and potassium related to

a. vomiting
b. dehydration

Ineffective family coping related to

a. hospitalization of infant
b. impending surgery for infant
c. knowledge deficit about medical diagnosis

Medical Diagnosis **PYLORIC STENOSIS, POSTOPERATIVE**

Primary Nursing Diagnosis **ALTERATION IN NUTRITION: LESS THAN BODY REQUIREMENTS**

Definition Insufficient (or infant is at risk of having insufficient) nutrients to meet body needs

Possibly Related to Postoperative vomiting

Characteristics Failure of bowel sounds to return
Inability to tolerate oral feedings

Expected Outcomes Infant will be adequately nourished as evidenced by

a. having a patent IV line that will deliver the ordered amount of IV fluids (state specific amount for each infant)
b. absorbing adequate amount of calories (state specific amount for each infant)
c. lack of
   —weight loss
   —vomiting when oral feedings are started

Possible Nursing Interventions

Keep accurate record of intake and output.

Assess and record IV fluids and condition of IV site every hour.

Keep infant elevated in a semi-erect position (use an infant seat).

Feed infant small amounts slowly with the infant in a semi-erect position.

Advance amount and type of feeding (as ordered) as infant tolerates.

Bubble infant before and frequently during feedings.

Organize care in order to decrease disturbing and handling infant after feedings.

Weigh infant daily on same scale at same time without clothes.

Evaluation for Charting

State intake and output.

Describe condition of IV site.

Was infant kept in a semi-erect position?

Were oral feedings tolerated?

State weight and determine if it is an increase or decrease from previous weight.

Related Nursing Diagnoses

Alteration in comfort: pain related to

a. surgical incision
b. hunger
c. vomiting and effect on operative site

Potential for infection related to

a. surgical incision
b. young age of patient
c. IV site

Ineffective family coping related to

a. having a young infant in the hospital
b. fear of the surgery not being successful

Medical Diagnosis **RENAL FAILURE, ACUTE**

Primary Nursing Diagnosis **ALTERATION IN FLUID AND ELECTROLYTE BALANCE***

Definition Disturbance in the amount of body fluid and disturbance in the values of body electrolytes

Possibly Related to
Decreased renal perfusion
Renal parenchymal injury or disease
Obstruction of renal system

Characteristics
Oliguria
Decreased urinary output
Edema
Hypertension
Tachypnea
Congestive heart failure
Diuresis
Hyperkalemia
Hyponatremia
Hypocalcemia
Metabolic acidosis

Expected Outcomes
Child will regain an adequate fluid volume and electrolyte balance as evidenced by

a. adequate urinary output (state specific highest and lowest outputs for each child)
b. receiving only the ordered amount of fluid intake (state exact amount allowed for each child)
c. lack of edema
d. normal blood pressure (state specific highest and lowest pressures for each child)

---

*Not NANDA approved at publication

e. serum potassium between 3.5 and 5.0 mEq/liter
f. serum sodium between 138 and 145 mEq/liter
g. serum chloride between 101 and 108 mEq/liter
h. serum carbon dioxide content between 18 and 27 mEq/liter

Possible Nursing Interventions

Keep accurate record of intake and output.

Assess and record

- signs/symptoms of renal failure (such as those listed under Characteristics) every 2 hours and prn
- laboratory values as indicated
- vital signs, including blood pressure every 2 hours and prn
- signs/symptoms of hyperkalemia including weakness, paralysis, numbness and tingling sensation, EKG changes, and cardiac dysrhythmias every 2 hours and prn

Evaluation for Charting

State intake and output.

State current laboratory values.

State range of vital signs including blood pressure.

Were any signs/symptoms of hyperkalemia noted?

Related Nursing Diagnoses

Decreased cardiac output related to

a. hypertension
b. edema

Alteration in nutrition: less than body requirements related to increased tissue catabolism

Potential for infection related to

a. invasive monitoring
b. poor systemic perfusion
c. poor nutritional state

Ineffective family coping related to the seriousness and emergency nature of the disease

Medical Diagnosis

REYE'S SYNDROME

Primary Nursing Diagnosis

ALTERATION IN LEVEL OF CONSCIOUSNESS*

Definition

Reduced or impaired state of awareness; can range from mild to complete impairment (coma)

Possibly Related to

Increased intracranial pressure

Characteristics

Antecedent viral infection
Vomiting
Change in level of consciousness
Irritability
Lethargy
Combative behavior
Hyperventilation
Positive Babinski sign
Pupillary changes
Coma
Abnormal posturing
Seizures

Expected Outcomes

Child will be free of signs/symptoms of increased intracranial pressure as evidenced by

a. lack of
   —vomiting
   —decorticate or decerebrate posturing
   —lethargy, extreme irritability, or combative behavior
   —seizures
b. respiratory rate within acceptable range (state specific highest and lowest rates for each child)
c. negative Babinski sign

---

*Not NANDA approved at publication

d. pupils that are equal and react to light
e. being alert and oriented when awake
f. intracranial pressure 15 to 20 mmHg

Possible Nursing Interventions

Assess and record at least 2 hours and prn

- neuro vital signs with regular vital signs
- signs/symptoms of increased intracranial pressure (see Characteristics)

Monitor intracranial pressure every 15 minutes. Notify physician if above 20 mmHg. Calculate and record cerebral perfusion pressure (mean arterial pressure minus intracranial pressure) every hour and prn.

Turn gently and slowly every 2 hours (side, back, side)

Elevate head of bed 30°; maintain head in midline position.

If intracranial catheter is in place, monitor intracranial pressure while suctioning patient. Hyperventilate patient if intracranial pressure increases above 20 mmHg; notify physician.

Keep environment as quiet as possible.

Organize nursing care to decrease disturbing and stimulating patient.

Keep accurate record of intake and output.

Evaluation for Charting

State results of neuro vital signs.

State any signs/symptoms of increased intracranial pressure. State any successful measures used to decrease intracranial pressure.

State highest and lowest respiratory rates.

State highest and lowest intracranial pressures.

Was head of bed maintained at 30° with head in midline position?

State intake and output.

Related Nursing Diagnoses

Impaired gas exchange related to

a. hyperventilation
b. increased intracranial pressure

Alteration in electrolyte balance: sodium and potassium related to

a. vomiting
b. hyperventilation
c. liver dysfunction

Fluid volume deficit related to

a. vomiting
b. hyperventilation (insensible water loss)

Alteration in nutrition: less than body requirements related to liver dysfunction

Ineffective family coping related to

a. sudden serious illness of child, possible death
b. multiple treatments and procedures
c. guilt from not having recognized symptoms as serious earlier
d. uncertain prognosis and sequelae

Medical Diagnosis **SALICYLATE POISONING**

Primary Nursing Diagnosis **IMPAIRED GAS EXCHANGE**

Definition Alteration in the exchange of oxygen and carbon dioxide in the lungs and/or at the cellular level

Possibly Related to Increase in the depth and rate of respirations resulting from the effect of the drug on the respiratory center

Characteristics
Hyperventilation
Hyperpyrexia
Diaphoresis
Vomiting
Diarrhea
Confusion
Lethargy
Coma

Expected Outcomes Child will have adequate gas exchange as evidenced by

a. clear and equal breath sounds
b. respiratory rate within normal range (state specific highest and lowest rates for each child)
c. arterial pH between 7.35 and 7.45
d. P_aCO_2 between 35 and 45 mmHg
e. P_aO_2 between 75 and 100 mmHg
f. arterial bicarbonate level between 22 and 28 mEq/liter
g. lack of signs/symptoms of respiratory alkalosis such as confusion, loss of consciousness, coma

Possible Nursing Interventions

Assess and record

- breath sounds every hour and prn; notify physician if respiratory rate is out of the acceptable range
- blood gas values when indicated and report any abnormalities to the physician
- signs/symptoms of alkalosis (such as those listed under Expected Outcome) every 2 hours and prn

Administer oxygen in the correct amount and route if ordered.

Evaluation for Charting

Describe breath sounds.

State highest and lowest respiratory rates.

State highest and lowest blood gas values, and determine the on-going physiologic process.

Describe any signs/symptoms of respiratory alkalosis noted.

State amount and route of oxygen delivery administered. State any improvement noted as a result of oxygen therapy.

Acute Related Nursing Diagnoses

Altered metabolic function related to

a. the accumulation of lactic acid
b. vomiting

Fluid volume deficit related to

a. vomiting
b. diarrhea
c. increased insensible water loss from rapid respirations

d. hyperpyrexia
e. diaphoresis

Decreased cardiac output related to

a. possible bleeding tendencies resulting from salicylate inhibition of platelet aggregation and prothrombin production
b. fluid volume deficit

Ineffective family coping related to

a. accidental illness of child
b. fear of child not recovering from ingestion
c. guilt from the circumstances of the child's illness
d. suicide attempt

Knowledge deficit, parental/family related to prevention and safety

Alteration in thermoregulation related to hyperpyrexia

Medical Diagnosis

SCOLIOSIS, POSTOPERATIVE

Primary Nursing Diagnosis

ALTERATION IN TISSUE PERFUSION

Definition

Potential for inadequate amount of blood and oxygen being delivered to the tissues in the body

Possibly Related to

Surgical procedure
Immobility
Bleeding bone
Shift in thoracic content
Pressure redistribution within the vascular system

Characteristics

Tachypnea
Rales, rhonchi
Unequal or diminished chest expansion
Irritability
Restlessness
Cyanosis

Expected Outcomes

Child will have an adequate amount of blood and oxygen being delivered to the tissues as evidenced by

a. respiratory rate within acceptable range (state specific highest and lowest rates for each child)
b. clear and equal breath sounds bilaterally
c. equal and adequate chest expansion
d. lack of
   —extreme irritability and restlessness
   —cyanosis

Possible Nursing Interventions

Assess and record any signs/symptoms of alteration in tissue perfusion (such as those listed under Characteristics).

Log roll child gently as ordered (usually every 2 hours). Obtain assistance when indicated.

Administer pain medication as ordered. Chart effectiveness.

Assess, record, and change dressing as ordered.

Evaluation for Charting

Describe any signs/symptoms of alteration of tissue perfusion noted and action taken if alteration was present.

Was child log rolled every 2 hours? Describe how child tolerated this procedure.

Describe amount and characteristics of pain and effectiveness of any pain medication given.

Describe surgical incision if dressing change was indicated. Describe amount and characteristics of any drainage noted on dressing.

Related Nursing Diagnoses

Alteration in comfort: pain related to surgical incision and repair

Decreased cardiac output related to

a. blood loss
b. extensive dissection and bleeding bone

Self-care deficit related to surgical repair and immobility

Impaired physical mobility related to surgical repair

Ineffective family coping related to

a. hospitalization of child
b. parental guilt from possible familial tendency of the defect

Disturbance in self-concept: body image related to

a. casting
b. insertion of rod or wires
c. stiff posture
d. scar

Medical Diagnosis

SEIZURE DISORDER

Primary Nursing Diagnosis

ALTERATION IN LEVEL OF CONSCIOUSNESS*

Definition Reduced or impaired state of awareness

Possibly Related to Seizure activity resulting from

- trauma
- infection
- degenerative neurologic disease
- metabolic disturbance
- electrolyte disturbance
- tumor
- fever

Characteristics Blinking

Lip smacking

Tonic-clonic movements

"Staring into space"

Tremors

Flaccidity

Sudden and uncontrollable onset of activity

Loss of consciousness

Can be preceded by an aura

Could be followed by a postictal state that can include drowsiness and confusion

Expected Outcome Child will be free of seizure activity.

Possible Nursing Interventions Assess for any early signs/symptoms (e.g., onset of uncontrollable activity or an aura) that may lead to seizure activity.

*Not NANDA approved at publication

Assess and record

- temperature; if elevated, check every hour
- all seizure activity including
  —beginning and progression sequence
  —duration
  —type of tremor
  —level of consciousness
  —incontinence

If seizure does occur

- stay with child
- protect head from injury
- try to gently insert padded tongue blade if child has not clamped down
- keep side rails up and padded if child is in bed
- move sharp objects away from child
- loosen any constrictive clothing at neck

Ensure antiseizure medications are administered on schedule. Assess for any side effects such as drowsiness, fatigue, and gastrointestinal upset.

Evaluation for Charting

Describe seizure activity, sequence, timing; aura or postictal phase.
State highest and lowest temperatures.
Were antiseizure medications given on schedule? Describe any side effects noted.

Related Nursing Diagnoses

Impaired gas exchange related to possible anoxia during seizure activity
Potential for injury related to seizure activity

Ineffective family coping related to

a. fear of child dying during a seizure
b. fear of child being injured during a seizure
c. fear of child being permanently brain damaged as the result of seizure activity
d. underlying disorder

Medical Diagnosis

SICKLE CELL CRISES

Primary Nursing Diagnosis

ALTERATION IN TISSUE PERFUSION

Definition

Inadequate amount of blood and oxygen being delivered to the tissues in the body

Possibly Related to

Anemia
Sickled red blood cells
Tissue hypoxia/ischemia

Characteristics

Anemia
Weakness
Fatigue
Anorexia
Pain in bones, joints, abdomen
Swelling of the hands and feet
Fever
Jaundice

Expected Outcomes

Child's tissues will have adequate supply of blood and oxygen as evidenced by

a. normal hemoglobin (state specific range for each child)
b. normal hematocrit (state specific range for each child)
c. warm, edema-free extremities
d. lack of discoloration of extremities
e. adequate fluid intake (state specific amount needed for each child)

Possible Nursing Interventions

Keep accurate record of intake and output.

Assess and record

- signs/symptoms of decreased tissue oxygenation (such as those

listed under Characteristics) every 2 hours and prn
- laboratory values as indicated

Give blood products as ordered. Assess, record, and report any signs/symptoms of transfusion reaction (e.g., chills, fever, headache, flank pain, urticaria, flushing, chest pain, difficulty breathing, irregular heart rate, apprehension).

Evaluation for Charting

State intake and output.

Describe any signs/symptoms of decreased tissue oxygenation noted.

State type and amount of any blood products given and state post-transfusion laboratory values. Describe any signs/symptoms of transfusion reaction noted.

Related Nursing Diagnoses

Potential for infection related to

a. anemia
b. fever

Decreased cardiac output related to anemia.

Alteration in comfort: pain related to joint, bone, or abdominal pain

Impaired physical mobility related to

a. fatigue
b. need to decrease oxygen requirements
c. tissue hypoxia

Ineffective family coping related to

a. long-term illness and uncertain prognosis
b. parental guilt due to genetic nature of the disease

Medical Diagnosis

TRACHEOESOPHAGEAL FISTULA, PREOPERATIVE

Primary Nursing Diagnosis

INEFFECTIVE AIRWAY CLEARANCE

Definition

Inability to adequately clear secretions from the airways

Possibly Related to

Congenital anomaly

Characteristics

Respiratory difficulty
Excessive amounts of mucus
Choking
Regurgitation
Coughing
Cyanosis, particularly at feeding time
Abdominal distention
Unsuccessful attempt to pass NG tube (if esophageal atresia is present)

Expected Outcomes

Infant will be able to clear airway adequately as evidenced by

a. clear and equal breath sounds
b. respiratory rate between 30 and 60 breaths/minute
c. lack of
—respiratory difficulty
—choking, coughing, and regurgitation (infant may need to be npo to accomplish this goal)
—abdominal distention

Possible Nursing Interventions

Assess and record breath sounds every 2 hours and prn.

Observe infant continuously during feedings for signs/symptoms of respiratory problems or keep npo.

Ensure mouth and nasopharynx are suctioned as ordered (sometimes continuously, sometimes intermittently). Assess characteristics of secretions.

Give humidified oxygen, if ordered, in the correct amount and by the correct route.

Keep accurate record of intake and output.

Evaluation for Charting

Describe breath sounds.

State highest and lowest respiratory rates.

If feedings were given, describe how infant tolerated feedings.

Describe characteristics of secretions.

If oxygen was ordered, state whether infant received the correct amount by the correct route and describe effect of oxygen therapy.

State intake and output.

Related Nursing Diagnoses

Fluid volume deficit related to

a. respiratory difficulty
b. excessive losses
c. inability to take oral fluids

Alteration in nutrition: less than body requirements related to

a. inability of infant to tolerate oral feedings
b. respiratory difficulty

Potential for infection related to

a. young age of patient
b. aspiration of fluid

Ineffective family coping related to

a. birth of an imperfect infant
b. need for infant to have surgery

Medical Diagnosis

TRACHEOESOPHAGEAL FISTULA, POSTOPERATIVE

Primary Nursing Diagnosis

INEFFECTIVE AIRWAY CLEARANCE

Definition

Inability to adequately clear secretions from the airway

Possibly Related to

Postoperative complications

Characteristics

Lack of patent airway
Increased pulmonary secretions
Improper functioning of chest tubes

Expected Outcomes

Infant will be able to clear airway adequately as evidenced by

a. clear and equal breath sounds
b. respiratory rate between 30 and 60 breaths/minute
c. lack of
   —retractions
   —cyanosis
d. correctly functioning chest tubes

Possible Nursing Interventions

Assess and record breath sounds every 2 hours and prn.

Assess and record any signs/symptoms of respiratory distress (e.g., rales, rhonchi, retractions, cyanosis) every 2 hours and prn.

Suction infant as needed. Be careful not to insert suction catheter too near the operative site (record correct length of catheter at the time of surgery).

Assess functioning of chest tubes every 30 minutes and record drainage as indicated. Strip (or milk) chest tubes as indicated if ordered.

Administer oxygen, if ordered, in the correct amount and by the correct route.

Administer NG suction/decompression if ordered. If NG tube becomes dislodged or comes out, do not reinsert (danger of disruption to suture line). Notify physician.

Evaluation for Charting

Describe breath sounds.

State highest and lowest respiratory rates.

Describe any signs/symptoms of respiratory difficulty noted.

Describe characteristics of secretions.

Describe characteristics of chest tube drainage.

If oxygen was ordered, state the amount and route of delivery administered. Describe effectiveness of therapy.

If NG tube is in place, state amount and characteristics of drainage.

Related Nursing Diagnoses

Alteration in comfort: pain related to surgical procedure

Fluid volume deficit related to

a. inability to take oral feedings
b. potential for respiratory difficulty
c. postoperative complications

Potential for infection related to

a. surgical procedure
b. invasive procedures (e.g., IV, chest tubes)
c. presurgical condition

Ineffective family coping related to

a. hospitalization of infant
b. discomfort infant may be experiencing

c. necessary monitoring equipment connected to infant
d. guilt regarding cause of defect

Section II: Pediatric Care Plans
B. Additional Nursing Diagnoses

Primary Nursing Diagnosis — **ALTERATION IN BOWEL ELIMINATION: CONSTIPATION**

Definition

Difficulty (or child is at risk for having difficulty) in passing stools; infrequent hard stools

Possibly Related to

Congenital anomaly
Postoperative complication
Immobility
Lack of time and/or privacy
Lack of adequate diet
Lack of adequate fluid intake

Characteristics

Hard infrequent stools
Abdominal distention
Decreased appetite
Headache
Feeling of rectal fullness
Pain and straining with bowel movement

Expected Outcomes

Child will have normal bowel elimination as evidenced by

a. normal type and number of bowel movements (specify for each child)
b. lack of
 —abdominal distention
 —decreased appetite
 —headache
 —feeling of rectal fullness
 —pain and straining with bowel movements

Possible Nursing Interventions

Assess and record number and characteristics of stools every shift.

Assess and record any signs/symptoms of constipation (such as those listed under Characteristics) every shift.

Keep accurate record of intake and output.

Encourage child to drink fruit juices if appropriate

Ensure child drinks an adequate amount of oral fluids (specify for each child).

Assess for effectiveness of prescribed stool softeners or laxatives.

Assess child's diet and its impact on bowel activity.

Evaluation for Charting

Describe stools.

List any signs/symptoms of constipation noted.

If stool softeners or laxatives were administered, state effectiveness.

Describe child's appetite.

Primary Nursing Diagnosis ALTERATION IN COMFORT: PAIN

Definition A condition in which an individual experiences (or is at risk for experiencing) discomfort

Possibly Related to

Inflammation
Surgical incision
Fear
Anxiety
Treatments and procedures
Headache
Neck pain
Earache
Fever
Hunger
Chest pain
Joint, bone, or abdominal pain
Cough
Constipation
Burn wound

Characteristics

Verbal communication of discomfort
Constant crying unrelieved by usual comfort measures
Facial grimacing
Physical signs/symptoms

- tachycardia
- tachypnea/bradypnea
- increased blood pressure
- diaphoresis
- pupillary dilation

Guarding of painful area

Expected Outcomes

Child will be free of severe/constant discomfort as evidenced by

a. verbal communication of comfort
b. lack of constant crying

c. lack of facial expression of discomfort
d. heart rate within acceptable range (state specific highest and lowest rates for each child)
e. respiratory rate within acceptable range (state specific highest and lowest rates for each child)
f. blood pressure within acceptable range (state specific highest and lowest pressures for each child)
g. lack of
—diaphoresis
—dilated pupils
—guarding

Possible Nursing Interventions

Assess and record any signs/symptoms of discomfort (such as those listed under Characteristics) at least once/shift.

Handle any painful areas gently.

Ensure analgesics are administered if needed. Assess and chart effectiveness.

Encourage family members to stay and comfort child when possible.

Allow family members to participate in the care of the child when possible.

Use distraction measures (e.g., playing games, watching TV) when appropriate.

Ensure antipyretics are administered on schedule if child has fever and assess for effectiveness.

Evaluation for Charting

Describe any signs/symptoms of discomfort noted.

If analgesics or antipyretics were given, describe effectiveness.

Describe any successful measures used to reduce discomfort.

Primary Nursing Diagnosis

ALTERATION IN ELECTROLYTE BALANCE: SODIUM AND POTASSIUM*

Definition

A disturbance (or child is at risk for having a disturbance) in the value of the body's sodium and potassium

Possibly Related to

Sodium imbalance: losses

- gastrointestinal losses: diarrhea and vomiting
- medications: diuretics
- burn injury
- renal disease: severe nephritis

Sodium imbalance: excess

- dehydration
- deficient production of antidiuretic hormone
- increased secretion of adrenocortical steroids
- hypersecretion of aldosterone

Potassium imbalance: losses

- gastrointestinal losses: diarrhea, vomiting, and NG suctioning
- increased renal losses: diuretics
- malabsorption
- starvation

Potassium imbalance: excess

- burn injury
- renal failure
- adrenocortical insufficiency
- internal hemorrhage
- trauma
- excessive intake
- acidosis

Characteristics

Sodium deficit (hyponatremia)

---

*Not NANDA approved at publication

- weakness
- delirium
- seizures
- oliguria

Sodium excess (hypernatremia)

- edema
- weight gain
- hypertension
- decreased urinary output

Potassium deficit (hypokalemia)

- decreased muscle activity
- paresthesias
- tetany
- atony
- coma
- shallow respirations
- hypotension and rapid pulse
- EKG changes: flat T waves, peaked P wave
- cardiac arrest

Potassium excess (hyperkalemia)

- weakness
- tremors, twitching
- paresthesia
- paralysis
- anuria
- EKG changes: spiked T waves, flattened P wave
- ventricular dysrhythmias
- cardiac arrest

Expected Outcomes

Child will have adequate electrolyte balance as evidenced by

a. serum sodium between 138 and 145 mEq/liter
b. serum potassium between 3.5 and 5.0 mEq/liter
c. normal sinus rhythm

d. heart rate within acceptable range (state specific highest and lowest rates for each child)
e. blood pressure within acceptable range (state specific highest and lowest pressures for each child)
f. normal urinary output (state specific highest and lowest outputs for each child)
g. lack of edema
h. adequate fluid intake (state specific range for each child)
i. adequate caloric intake (state specific quantity for each child)
j. absence of signs/symptoms of hyponatremia, hypernatremia, hypokalemia, and hyperkalemia such as those listed under Characteristics

Possible Nursing Interventions

Assess and record vital signs every 2 hours and prn.

Keep accurate record of intake and output.

Assess and record any signs/symptoms of electrolyte imbalance (such as those listed under Characteristics) every 2 hours and prn. Report any abnormalities to the physician.

Assess and record laboratory values as indicated. Report abnormalities to the physician.

Instruct child/family in foods high and low in sodium and potassium.

Evaluation for Charting

State high and low range of vital signs.

State intake and output.

Describe any signs/symptoms of electrolyte imbalance noted.

State current laboratory values. If any were abnormal, state action taken and effectiveness or results of action taken.

Primary Nursing Diagnosis **ALTERATION IN PATTERNS OF URINARY ELIMINATION, RETENTION**

Definition Inability of the body to eliminate urine adequately

Possibly Related to

Decreased renal perfusion
Decreased cardiac output
Urinary tract anomalies
Renal infection
Neurogenic bladder
Side effects of antibiotic therapy

Characteristics

Decreased urinary output
Edema
Hypertension
Headache
Fever
Abdominal pain
Sudden weight gain

Expected Outcomes

Child will be free of urinary retention as evidenced by

a. adequate urinary output (state specific minimum amount for each child)
b. blood pressure within normal range (state specific highest and lowest pressures for each child)
c. lack of
—headache
—edema
—abdominal pain
d. return to regular body weight prior to illness

Possible Nursing Interventions

Keep accurate record of intake and output.

If child is on limited fluids, offer the correct amount to child on schedule.

Assess and record any signs/symptoms of urinary retention (such as those listed under Characteristics) at least every 8 hours.

Weigh child daily at same time of day using the same scale (nude or wearing underwear only).

Evaluation for Charting

State the child's intake and output.

State if child received the correct amount of fluid intake and how it was tolerated.

State any signs/symptoms of urinary retention noted.

State the child's weight and determine if it is an increase or decrease from the previous recorded weight.

Primary Nursing Diagnosis — **DEVELOPMENTAL DELAY***

Definition

Failure to progress (or the child is at risk for failure to progress) in expected tasks and skills (e.g., motor, feeling, sleep, play, language, and dressing) according to chronologic age

Possibly Related to

Increased intracranial pressure
Cerebral vascular infarcts
Brain abscess
Environmental problems (e.g., lack of stimulation)
Nutritional deficit
Parental knowledge deficit
Repeated or long-term hospitalization
Chronic or terminal illness

Characteristics

Will vary with age and stage of development of each child (refer to a growth and development chart); for example, a normal 3-month-old would

- hold head up when placed on abdomen
- follow objects
- regard face of others
- smile responsively
- manifest Moro sucking and rooting reflexes

Expected Outcomes

Child will progress developmentally as evidenced by

a. lack of markedly regressed behavior
b. continuation of pre-illness activities

---

*Not NANDA approved at publication

Parents will describe specific tasks/skills child should be able to do.

Possible Nursing Interventions

Allow child to move around in bed/crib when possible.

If restraints are needed, remove restraints when child can be monitored constantly.

Put familiar washable articles, such as toys and favorite blanket, in the bed/crib with the child.

Play games with child or encourage family to play with child when possible.

For children who are school aged, assist in arranging for child to continue with school work when possible.

Assist family in helping child to progress developmentally by offering developmentally appropriate activities.

Encourage family to continue some limit setting on child's behavior while hospitalized so the child will feel secure.

Evaluation for Charting

Describe any developmental delays or regressed behavior noted.

Describe child's level of developmental tasks/skills attainment.

Primary Nursing Diagnosis — **DISTURBANCE IN SELF-CONCEPT: BODY IMAGE**

Definition A condition in which the child has a negative view (or is at risk for having a negative view) of self

Possibly Related to

Edema
Loss of body part(s)
Present and/or future scar tissue
Contractures

Characteristics

Verbalization about displeasure in body
Refusal to look into mirror
Refusal to participate in care
Decreased interest in appearance
Loss of interest in usual activities (e.g., visiting with friends, talking on the phone)

Expected Outcomes

Child will indicate acceptance of body image as evidenced by

a. ability to look in mirror
b. willingness to participate in care
c. developmentally appropriate interest in appearance
d. ability to carry on with usual activities
e. verbalization of a positive body image

Possible Nursing Interventions

Assess and record child's and/or family's ability to accept altered body image.
Encourage child and/or family to look at altered body area and express their feelings and concerns.
Encourage child and/or family to participate in care when possible.
Encourage child to carry on with usual activities.

Evaluation for Charting

Describe child's and/or family's ability to accept altered body image.

Describe any successful methods used that helped child and/or family cope with child's altered body image.

Was child and/or family able to look at altered body area?

Was child and/or family willing to participate in care?

Did child show appropriate interest in his/her appearance?

Did child participate in usual activities?

Primary Nursing Diagnosis: FEAR, CHILD'S

Definition

Feeling of apprehension (or the child is at risk for having feelings of apprehension) resulting from a known source

Possibly Related to

Respiratory distress
Unfamiliar surroundings
Forced contact with strangers
Treatments and procedures
Restraints
Hospitalization
Terminal illness
Knowledge deficit

Characteristics

Uncooperativeness
Regressed behavior
Restlessness
Verbalization of danger/fear
Constant crying
Tachypnea
Tachycardia
Diaphoresis

Expected Outcomes

Child will exhibit only a minimal amount of fear as evidenced by

a. relating appropriately to family members
b. being able to rest and sleep between treatments and procedures
c. lack of constant crying
d. respiratory rate within acceptable range (state specific highest and lowest rates for each child)
e. heart rate within acceptable range (state specific highest and lowest rates for each child)
f. lack of diaphoresis

Possible Nursing Interventions

Decrease child's fear when possible by

- encouraging family members to stay with child
- encouraging family members to participate in the care of the child
- trying to have the same staff members care for the child
- talking to child and explaining procedures and treatments along with rationale for why they are necessary
- trying to spend extra time with the child when the family members are unable to be present

Assess and record any physiologic signs/symptoms of fear (e.g., increased respiratory rate, increased heart rate, and diaphoresis) when taking vital signs.

Evaluation for Charting

State whether child manifested fear and describe any successful measures used to help alleviate the fear.

Does the child's fear decrease if family members stay and participate in the child's care?

State highest and lowest respiratory and heart rates.

Was diaphoresis present?

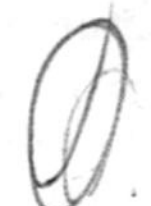

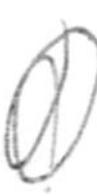

Primary Nursing Diagnosis

GUILT, PARENTAL/FAMILY

Definition

A state or condition in which the individual(s) accept(s) blame (or is at risk for accepting blame) either appropriate or inappropriate

Possibly Related to

Genetic nature of the disease
Delay in seeking health care
Neglect, abuse

Characteristics

Verbalization of blame
Overprotectiveness of ill child
Anger
Irritability

Expected Outcomes

Parents/family will be able to appropriately deal with guilt feelings as evidenced by

a. expressing fears/concerns to members of the health care team
b. participating in child's care when possible
c. accepting help when indicated

Possible Nursing Interventions

Allow and encourage family to ventilate and express feelings of guilt; give positive reinforcement for doing so.

Praise any positive observed family/child interactions.

Encourage family to participate in child's care when possible.

Encourage and assist family in seeking outside help/counseling when appropriate.

Evaluation for Charting

Describe any concerns/fears expressed by family.

Did family participate in child's care?

Describe any successful measures used to help decrease family's guilt feelings.

Did family seek outside counseling?

Primary Nursing Diagnosis: IMPAIRED PHYSICAL MOBILITY

Definition

Limited ability (or the child is at risk for limited ability) of movement

Possibly Related to

- Inflammation
- Fatigue
- Tissue hypoxia
- Increased oxygen requirements
- Decreased cardiac output
- Contractures
- Surgical repair
- Imposed restrictions as part of treatment for disease state
- Decreased muscle strength
- Paralysis, weakness
- Edema
- External device or equipment (e.g., casts, splints, braces, IV tubing)
- Pain

Characteristics

- Inability to move part or all of the body
- Inability to ambulate because of imposed restrictions (e.g., bedrest)
- Decreased range of motion
- Limited or decreased coordination

Expected Outcomes

Child will comply with imposed mobility limitations without extreme agitation as evidenced by appropriate age-related behaviors such as

a. playing in crib with toys
b. lack of constant crying
c. talking on the phone to friends and family
d. watching TV
e. reading
f. participating in care to the extent possible

g. accepting necessary treatments and procedures

Child will return to activity level prior to illness upon discharge.

Possible Nursing Interventions

Assess and record child's activity level at least once/shift.

Encourage family members to stay with child when possible.

Encourage and make available activities that the child can do within own limitations.

Arrange for play therapy, occupational therapy, and/or physical therapy when appropriate.

Evaluation for Charting

Describe child's current level of activity.

Were family members able to remain with child?

Describe any successful measures used to keep child entertained.

Was play therapy, occupational therapy, and/or physical therapy involved in child's care? If so, describe effectiveness of therapy and tolerance level of child.

Primary Nursing Diagnosis

POTENTIAL FOR INJURY

Definition

Situation in which child sustains (or is at risk for sustaining) damage or harm

Possibly Related to

Alteration in level of consciousness
Seizures
Accidents
Unsteady gait resulting in falls
Chemical dependency
Medication overdose/poisoning
Developmental level

Characteristics

Altered level of consciousness
Altered behavior
Fatigue
Pain
Open wounds
Hemorrhage
Pupillary changes
Swelling, edema

Expected Outcome

Child will be free of injury.

Possible Nursing Interventions

Keep side rails up on young children and those who are at risk for sustaining an injury.

Always have toddlers completely supervised by a staff or family member when out of bed.

Keep sharp or harmful objects out of reach of young children.

Always position infants on the abdomen, side, and/or in the head-elevated position after feedings.

Instruct family members not to prop bottles for infants (explain rationale).

Provide developmentally appropriate anticipatory guidance about safety.

Evaluation for Charting

Were side rails kept up?

Were toddlers supervised when out of bed?

Describe infant's position after feedings.

Describe any successful measures used to decrease injury to child.

Primary Nursing Diagnosis

SELF-CARE DEFICIT

Definition

Inability (or potential for inability) of child to maintain activities of daily living such as feeding, bathing, dressing, and toileting without partial or complete assistance

Possibly Related to

Postoperative surgical limitations
Accident or injury limitations
Disease process imposing limitations
Altered level of consciousness
Pain
Depression

Characteristics

Inability to feed self unassisted
Inability to bathe self unassisted
Inability to dress self unassisted
Inability to take care of toileting needs unassisted

Expected Outcome

Child will be able to either completely or partially take care of developmentally appropriate activities of daily living.

Possible Nursing Interventions

Encourage and assist child to perform as many activities of daily living as possible. This may require cutting up food so child can feed self. Provide appropriate utensils such as spoon (instead of fork) or cup with a large handle.

Encourage family members to participate in care of child when possible.

Demonstrate alternative methods of accomplishing tasks such as moving in bed, getting in and out of bed, dressing and feeding self.

Be sure call bell is always within child's reach.

Keep side rails up at all times if indicated.

Praise child for any success achieved.

Assist child and family in obtaining special devices, such as electric toothbrush, that will help child perform activities of daily living.

Evaluation for Charting

Describe extent of child's self-care deficit.

Did family participate in care?

Was call bell kept within child's reach?

Were side rails kept up?

Were any special devices needed? If so, were they effective in helping child to perform activities of daily living?

Reference List

Carpenito, L. (1985). *Handbook of nursing diagnosis*. Philadelphia: Lippincott.

Gordon, M. (1985). *Manual of nursing diagnosis 1984-1985*. New York: McGraw-Hill.

Index

Caffeine 10mg/kg loading
2.5mg/kg maintenance

5mg/kg Gent loading
4mg/kg
2.5mg/kg preemie